D1585584

Urgent Care Emergencies

Avoiding the Pitfalls and Improving the Outcomes

LIBRARY
POOLE HOSPITAL
POOLE
BH15 2JB
TEL: 01202 442101
PGMC.library@poole.nhs.uk

Urgent Care Emergencies

Avoiding the Pitfalls and Improving the Outcomes

EDITED BY

Deepi G. Goyal, MD

Associate Professor
Department of Emergency Medicine
Mayo Clinic, College of Medicine
Rochester, MN
USA

Amal Mattu, MD, FAAEM, FACEP

Professor and Vice Chair
Director, Faculty Development Fellowship
Department of Emergency Medicine
University of Maryland School of Medicine
Baltimore, MD
USA

WILEY-BLACKWELL

A John Wiley & Sons, Ltd., Publication

This edition first published 2012, © 2012 by John Wiley & Sons, Ltd.

Wiley-Blackwell is an imprint of John Wiley & Sons, formed by the merger of Wiley's global Scientific, Technical and Medical business with Blackwell Publishing.

Registered Office
John Wiley & Sons, Ltd, The Atrium, Southern Gate, Chichester, West Sussex, PO19 8SQ, UK

Editorial Offices
9600 Garsington Road, Oxford, OX4 2DQ, UK
The Atrium, Southern Gate, Chichester, West Sussex, PO19 8SQ, UK
111 River Street, Hoboken, NJ 07030-5774, USA

For details of our global editorial offices, for customer services and for information about
how to apply for permission to reuse the copyright material in this book please see our website
at www.wiley.com/wiley-blackwell.

The right of the author to be identified as the author of this work has been asserted in accordance with the UK Copyright, Designs and Patents Act 1988.

All rights reserved. No part of this publication may be reproduced, stored in a retrieval system, or transmitted, in any form or by any means, electronic, mechanical, photocopying, recording or otherwise, except as permitted by the UK Copyright, Designs and Patents Act 1988, without the prior permission of the publisher.

Designations used by companies to distinguish their products are often claimed as trademarks. All brand names and product names used in this book are trade names, service marks, trademarks or registered trademarks of their respective owners. The publisher is not associated with any product or vendor mentioned in this book. This publication is designed to provide accurate and authoritative information in regard to the subject matter covered. It is sold on the understanding that the publisher is not engaged in rendering professional services. If professional advice or other expert assistance is required, the services of a competent professional should be sought.

Library of Congress Cataloging-in-Publication Data

Urgent care emergencies : avoiding the pitfalls and improving the outcomes / edited by Deepi G. Goyal, Amal Mattu.
       p. ; cm.
  Includes bibliographical references and index.
  ISBN 978-0-470-65772-0 (pbk. : alk. paper)
I. Goyal, Deepi.   II. Mattu, Amal.
[DNLM: 1. Ambulatory Care.   2. Emergencies.   3. Treatment Outcome.   WB 101]
   362.12–dc23
                                                 2012008537

A catalogue record for this book is available from the British Library.

Wiley also publishes its books in a variety of electronic formats. Some content that appears in print may not be available in electronic books.

Set in 9/12 pt Meridien by SPi Publisher Services, Pondicherry, India

Printed in Singapore by Ho Printing Singapore Pte Ltd

1   2012

Contents

List of Contributors

Michael K. Abraham, MD, MS
Clinical Assistant Professor
Department of Emergency Medicine
University of Maryland School of
Medicine
Baltimore, MD, USA

Christopher E. Anderson, MD
Resident Physician
Department of Emergency Medicine
Mayo Clinic
Rochester, MN, USA

Jana L. Anderson, MD
Instructor of Emergency Medicine
Division of Emergency Medicine
Research
Mayo Clinic
Rochester, MN, USA

Eric T. Boie, MD, FAAEM
Assistant Professor of Emergency
Medicine
Department of Emergency Medicine
Mayo Clinic
Rochester, MN, USA

Michael C. Bond, MD
Assistant Professor
Department of Emergency Medicine
University of Maryland School of
Medicine
Baltimore, MD, USA

Ronna L. Campbell, MD, PhD
Assistant Professor of Emergency
Medicine
Department of Emergency Medicine
Mayo Clinic
Rochester, MN, USA

Nadia Eltaki, MD
Resident Physician
Department of Emergency Medicine
University of Maryland Medical Center
Baltimore, MD, USA

Alisa M. Gibson, MD, DMD
Clinical Assistant Professor
Department of Emergency Medicine
University of Maryland School of
Medicine
Baltimore, MD, USA

James L. Homme, MD
Consultant Pediatrics and Emergency
Medicine
Mayo Clinic
Rochester, MN, USA

Christopher S. Kiefer, MD
Assistant Professor of Clinical
Emergency Medicine
Indiana University School of Medicine
Indianapolis, IN, USA

Hyung T. (Henry) Kim, MD
Assistant Professor of Clinical
Emergency Medicine
University of Southern California
Los Angeles County Hospital
Los Angeles, CA, USA

Michael J. Laughlin, Jr., MD
Instructor of Emergency Medicine
Mayo Clinic College of Medicine
Rochester, MN, USA

Jennifer A. Lisowe, MD, FAAD
Department of Dermatology
Mayo Clinic Health System
Owatonna, MN, USA

**Joseph P. Martinez, MD, FACEP,
FAAEM**
Assistant Professor of Emergency
Medicine
Assistant Dean for Student Affairs
University of Maryland School of
Medicine
Baltimore, MD, USA

Siamak Moayedi, MD
Assistant Professor, Department of
Emergency Medicine
University of Maryland School of
Medicine
Baltimore, MD, USA

David M. Nestler, MD, MS
Assistant Professor of Emergency
Medicine
Division of Emergency Medicine
Research
Mayo Clinic College of Medicine
Rochester, MN, USA

Stephen M. Schenkel, MD, MPP
Associate Professor
Department of Emergency Medicine
University of Maryland School of
Medicine
Baltimore, MD;
Chief, Emergency Medicine
Mercy Medical Center
Baltimore, MD, USA

Sarah K. Sommerkamp, MD
Assistant Professor
Department of Emergency Medicine
University of Maryland School of
Medicine
Baltimore, MD, USA

Mercedes Torres, MD
Clinical Assistant Professor
Department of Emergency Medicine
University of Maryland School of
Medicine
Baltimore, MD, USA

Reinier van Tonder, MD
Clinical Instructor in Emergency
Medicine
Department of Emergency Medicine
Kaiser Permanente
San Diego Medical Center
San Diego, CA, USA

Brooks M. Walsh, MD
Attending Physician
Bridgeport Hospital,
Yale New Haven Health System,
Bridgeport, CT, USA

George Willis, MD
Clinical Assistant Professor
Department of Emergency Medicine
University of Maryland School of
Medicine;
Attending Physician
Mercy Medical Center
Baltimore, MD, USA

Preface

Healthcare systems are under stress. Many systems lack the capacity to manage the increasing volume of patients requiring care. Simultaneously, healthcare costs are under increased scrutiny by both fundors and providers, and they must be managed carefully to keep those systems sustainable. Traditional emergency departments and accident wards are becoming increasingly overcrowded and costly; and on the other hand primary care providers are often working at capacity or unavailable after hours. Consequently, patients with acute but minor illnesses are facing increasing challenges regarding where to obtain prompt medical care.

Urgent care centers were borne out of the need for practitioners and facilities that could provide access to individuals with noncritical illness and injuries to receive episodic, unscheduled care. Also known as fast tracks, walk-in centers, or minor injury units, these facilities are in high demand. They have a practitioner (physician, nurse practitioner, or physician assistant) on site during hours of operation and most have on-site x-ray, phlebotomy, and the capability to perform minor procedures.

Urgent care centers serve an important role in improving access to care for patients with noncritical injuries and illnesses. Furthermore, by caring for patients with lower acuity complaints, they allow already overcrowded emergency departments to provide care for higher acuity patients requiring their resources.

Though seemingly minor, some injuries and illnesses can have devastating consequences if not identified early or if managed incorrectly. Patients can be neither assumed nor expected to be able to differentiate a minor from a serious condition. Yet an unidentified orthopedic injury, improperly managed wound, or misidentified rash could have dire and long-lasting consequences. Practitioners must therefore always be on guard to ensure optimal care.

This text was developed to help providers who evaluate low acuity complaints in any setting. The aim is to highlight common pitfalls in the management of these seemingly low-acuity conditions. This text is not meant to be comprehensive in scope; rather it is meant to bring the provider's attention to high-risk aspects of chief complaints that may be encountered in these low-acuity settings.

The authors for each chapter were carefully chosen for having expertise in their respective topics, and have focused their chapters on high-risk pitfalls in everyday practice. At the end of each chapter, the authors have provided important pearls of wisdom for improving patient outcomes. The text is intended for any practitioner who cares for patients with these complaints – whether in an emergency department, an urgent care center, or any other healthcare setting. The text is designed to be of an appropriate size and practicality to be read cover-to-cover and to be used frequently during daily practice. On behalf of all of the authors, we sincerely hope that the pages that follow help you in helping your patients.

Deepi G. Goyal
Rochester, MN
Amal Mattu
Baltimore, MD

CHAPTER 1

HEENT Pitfalls

Alisa M. Gibson and Sarah K. Sommerkamp
Department of Emergency Medicine, University of Maryland School of Medicine, Baltimore, MD, USA

Introduction

Emergencies affecting the ear, nose, and throat (ENT) constitute a large component of chief complaints seen in urgent care centers. The majority of these patients have benign conditions that can be managed on an outpatient basis. Some seemingly innocuous complaints can be reflective of diseases that pose significant risk of morbidity and possibly mortality. As with most diseases, the key to differentiating between minor and dangerous conditions is the history and physical examination. A huge spectrum of pathology can manifest in the head and neck, and the management of this patient group can be overwhelming for an individual practitioner. In this chapter, we present key facts, highlight the pitfalls inherent in diagnosing these conditions, and offer pearls intended to facilitate their management.

Eye

Pitfall | Failure to ensure that patients with epithelial defects are treated with appropriate antibiotics and seen by an ophthalmologist within 24 hours

A wide variety of eye complaints are encountered by acute care providers. Differentiation between corneal abrasions, corneal ulcers, and corneal foreign bodies can be difficult. The majority of patients with any of these conditions present with eye pain and a gritty or foreign body sensation. Visual acuity may be affected, depending on the location of the defect, so testing and documenting visual acuity are essential, as they are in all patients with eye complaints. Acute monocular visual loss may signify a more dangerous condition, such as central retinal artery occlusion, central retinal vein occlusion, acute angle closure glaucoma, or retinal detachment or a central nervous process (stroke, transient ischemic attack (TIA), or multiple sclerosis (MS)). Patients with any of these signs should be referred to an emergency department.

Patients with suspected corneal epithelial defects should have a full eye examination. A slit lamp is preferred to Wood's lamp. The instillation of analgesic and/or cycloplegic drops will significantly relieve the patient's symptoms and increased his/her ability to tolerate the examination, but these drops should not be used if globe rupture is suspected. Fluorescein staining is mandatory for the evaluation of a corneal defect and to rule out herpes keratitis. Defects in the epithelial surface appear as a stain that does not clear with blinking. The size and position of any defect(s) should be documented. Punctate defects, which appear in a circular pattern, are sometimes seen in contact lens wearers, particularly after prolonged wear. Larger defects with a crater formation are ulcers.

Parallel vertical abrasions should raise suspicion for a foreign body under the lid. When this type of injury is detected, the patient's eyelid should be

Urgent Care Emergencies: Avoiding the Pitfalls and Improving the Outcomes, First Edition.
Edited by Deepi G. Goyal and Amal Mattu.
© 2012 John Wiley & Sons, Ltd. Published 2012 by John Wiley & Sons, Ltd.

Table 1.1 Treatment of corneal abrasions, ulcers, and foreign bodies

	Antibiotic	Ointment dose	Drops dose	Duration
No contacts	Trimethoprim/ polymyxin B	0.5″ four times a day	1–2 drops q 2 h	Continue until symptom free for >24 h
No contacts	Erythromycin	0.5″ q 3–4 h	None	Continue until symptom free for >24 h
No contacts	Sulfacetamide	0.5″ four times a day	1–3 drops q 2–3 h	Continue until symptom free for >24
Contacts	Tobramycin	0.5″ three times a day (severe infection, q 3–4 h)	1–2 drops q 4 h Severe infection: 2 drops q 30–60 min	Until evaluation by ophthalmology
Contacts	Ciprofloxacin	None	1–2 drops four times a day	Until evaluation by ophthalmology
Ulcer	Tobramycin	0.5″ q 3–4 h	2 drops q 30–60 min	Until evaluation by ophthalmology
Ulcer	Ciprofloxacin	None	1–2 drops q 1 h	Until evaluation by ophthalmology

Data from Silverman MA, Bessman E. Conjunctivitis: treatment and medication. Medscape. http://emedicine.medscape.com/article/797874-overview. April 27, 2010.

everted to allow further assessment. Without treatment, and over time, the vertical abrasions will coalesce and form an ulcer. Foreign bodies may also be lodged directly on the corneal surface. In many cases, they can be removed with a cotton swab or irrigation, but if that procedure is unsuccessful, removal with a needle or burr may be necessary and should be done only by someone with specific training. Metal foreign bodies may lead to the development of a rust ring, which should only be removed by an ophthalmologist [1].

> KEY FACT | **Foreign bodies or rust rings can wait up to 24 hours for removal by an ophthalmologist.**

The immediate treatment of corneal abrasions, ulcers, and foreign bodies is similar (Table 1.1). Simple abrasions that are smaller than 3 mm do not require follow-up as long as no foreign body is present, the patient's visual acuity is normal, and symptoms resolve within 24 hours [2]. However, if there is any doubt, referral to an ophthalmologist is reasonable. All other defects should be seen by a specialist within 24 hours. Antibiotics, which may be prescribed as either ointment or drops, should be administered to all patients with epithelial defects. Ointment is generally preferred (particularly for children) because it is easier to apply, stays in place longer, and lubricates

the eye. However, ointments are not well tolerated by most adults because they obscure vision and interfere with activities such as driving and reading. Drops are dispersed by the natural lubrication mechanisms of the eye. Firmly squeezing the eye shut for 5 minutes after administration will close the drainage ducts and increase penetration. Contact lens wearers with corneal abrasions require antipseudomonal antibiotic coverage and should be advised to refrain from wearing their contacts until they are cleared to do so by an ophthalmologist. All patients with corneal ulcers also require antipseudomonal antibiotic coverage.

Patients with painful corneal abrasion may require systemic narcotics. Ophthalmic nonsteroidal anti-inflammatory drugs (NSAIDs) may be prescribed, but are expensive. Topical anesthetics such as tetracaine should never be prescribed or given to patients for use at home, as repeated use may be associated with the development of ulcers. Tetanus status should be updated as needed. Eye patching has not been shown to be effective in accelerating healing. In fact, because it might worsen the infection and thus lengthen the time to recovery, it is not recommended [3].

> KEY FACT | **All patients with corneal ulcers require antipseudomonal antibiotic coverage.**

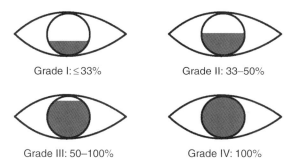

Grade I: ≤33%

Grade II: 33–50%

Grade III: 50–100%

Grade IV: 100%

Figure 1.1 Grades of hyphema.

Pitfall | **Failure to identify high-risk patients with hyphema who require inpatient admission**

A hyphema is a collection of blood in the anterior chamber. Patients typically present with eye pain and pupillary constriction. Visual acuity is variably affected, based on the amount of blood present. The condition most commonly results from trauma, but it can appear spontaneously in patients with sickle cell anemia or bleeding dyscrasias. Hyphemas are graded on a scale of I to IV, based on the amount of blood present (Figure 1.1). The hyphema grade is important to the clinical management and disposition of the patient. Visual acuity should be documented and globe rupture ruled out before a complete eye examination – including measurement of intraocular pressure – is performed. Concomitant ocular and bony injuries are common in patients with hyphema. Computed tomography (CT) may be indicated for patients with facial trauma. Laboratory studies to identify coagulopathy (complete blood count (CBC), prothrombin time (PT), partial thromboplastin time (PTT)) should be done in patients with known or suspected bleeding disorders. After globe rupture is excluded, ultrasound, if available, can be used to evaluate the eye for retinal detachment, lens damage, an intraocular foreign body, and choroidal hemorrhage [4].

All patients with hyphema are at risk of long-term complications such as synechiae and angle recession, cataracts, and delayed bleeding, and therefore must be followed up daily by an ophthalmologist. Certain patients have risk factors that necessitate emergent consultation and might warrant admission: these include sickle cell disease, bleeding dyscrasias (such as anticoagulation or hemophilia), potentially open globes, young age, and grade III or IV hyphemas [5–7]. Healthy compliant patients with none of the above risk factors who have hyphemas that fill less than 50% of the anterior chamber can be discharged home with ophthalmologic follow-up within 12 to 24 hours. Interventions are focused on an avoidance of re-bleeding and prevention of intraocular hypertension. Patients should be placed with the head of the bed elevated 30 degrees, in a dim quiet room. An eyeshield should be placed, and removed only for examination. The patient should be placed on bed rest with bathroom privileges and should not read or watch television as those activities may cause pupillary constriction and obstruct outflow. Analgesia with topical cycloplegics may be used, and systemic narcotics are frequently also required. NSAIDs should be avoided because of their associated bleeding risk. Nausea and vomiting should be treated aggressively since they can raise intraocular pressure. These instructions should be clearly communicated to any patient being discharged.

Throat

Sore throat is an extremely common complaint. It has a broad differential, ranging from viral illness to life-threatening conditions such as epiglottis and retropharyngeal abscess. In the majority of cases, these conditions can be differentiated by the history and physical examination. The fear of "strep throat" brings many people to acute care centers. Most people do not realize, however, that infection with Group A Streptococcus (GAS) is responsible for fewer than 10% of cases [8]. Other bacterial causes of acute pharyngitis include gonorrhea, diphtheria, and *Fusobacterium*. Viruses account for the majority of cases of pharyngitis. Typical viral pathogens include adenovirus, Epstein–Barr virus (EBV), cytomegalorvirus (CMV), the human immunodeficiency virus (HIV), and influenza.

> KEY FACT | **Viruses account for the majority of cases of pharyngitis. Group A Streptococcus is responsible for fewer than 10% of cases.**

Pitfall | Indiscriminate use of antibiotics for acute pharyngitis

Treatment of GAS pharyngitis with antibiotics can reduce the duration of illness by 1 or 2 days, decrease the risk of transmission, and prevent nonsuppurative complications (rheumatic fever and post-streptococcal glomerulonephritis, which are both rare among adults in the United States) and suppurative complications (peritonsillar abscess, sinusitis, retropharyngeal abscess). Those treatment goals, although well intentioned, lead to a great deal of prescriptions for unwarranted antibiotics. Overuse of antibiotics is typically thought of as hazardous to the population at large in terms of increasing resistance patterns, but it can also be dangerous for the individual. Disruption of the normal flora puts the patient at risk of superinfections by organisms such as *Candida* and *Clostridium difficile* and makes the antibiotic less effective for that patient for a full year [9]. The decision to prescribe antibiotics can be based on the individual patient's condition or by a combination of culture, the rapid streptococcal antigen test (RSAT), and the Centor criteria (see below). The use of culture is often impractical in an acute care practice, given that it can take 2 or 3 days to get results. The RSAT is 70–90% sensitive and 90–100% specific [10–12]. To perform this test, vigorously swab both tonsils and the posterior pharynx. Obtaining an adequate sample is crucial, as sensitivities correlate directly to inoculum size [13]. A positive test result is helpful, but a negative result does not rule out the disease. Many facilities do not have RSAT capabilities, so the diagnosis of GAS pharyngitis is frequently based on clinical criteria.

The Centor criteria constitute a clinical decision rule designed to assist with the diagnosis of streptococcal pharyngitis. The four criteria are tonsillar exudates, swollen, tender anterior cervical nodes, the absence of a cough, and a history of (or current) fever. If none of these criteria is present, the likelihood of a culture being positive for the presence of GAS is 2.5%. The likelihood of a positive test result increases with the number of criteria present: one criterion, 6.5%; two criteria, 15%; three criteria, 32%; and all four criteria, 56% [11]. The Centor criteria have a better negative than positive predictive value. Treatment based on the presence of three or four criteria alone will lead to overtreatment of 50%. The absence of three or four criteria leads to a negative predictive value of 80%, making this information more clinically useful.

> KEY FACT | **The presence of all four Centor criteria confers a risk of Group A Streptococcus pharyngitis of 56%**

Several studies have evaluated treatment strategies based on a combination of clinical criteria, RSAT, and culture, yielding variable results [14, 15]. The general recommendation is as follows: adults with fewer than two Centor criteria should not receive further testing or treatment. Adults with two or more criteria should be tested with RSAT, without reflex culture for negative results. Antibiotic treatment based on a positive RSAT is reasonable, but treatment based on clinical symptoms alone is not recommended [14, 16, 17]. Treatment recommendations for children differ, and a more generous treatment strategy can be adopted for adults in close contact with children. The traditional antibiotic regimen is penicillin, in either an intramuscular preparation (benzathine penicillin G, 1.2 million units given once) or an oral form (PenVK, 500 mg PO, BID for 10 days). Macrolides can be used for penicillin-allergic patients (azithromycin, 500 mg PO, daily for day 1, then 250 mg PO daily for days 2–5). Recent studies have shown improved bacterial eradication with cephalosporins, although this has not yet been proven to be clinically significant [18, 19].

Adjunctive treatment for GAS pharyngitis includes hydration, fever control, and in some cases corticosteroids. Several studies have shown that corticosteroids improve severe throat pain and shorten the clinical course [20–22]. Dexamethasone, 10 mg IV or IM, can be given as a one-time dose, making it convenient. Alternatively, prednisone can be prescribed as a 5-day, 40-mg burst. Analgesia with acetaminophen, NSAIDs, or topical numbing medications may be used. Patients with a strep throat can generally be discharged, providing they can tolerate fluid.

> KEY FACT | **Corticosteroids improve severe throat pain and shorten the clinical course of GAS pharyngitis**

Mononucleosis deserves special consideration for any patient with pharyngitis, particularly if antibiotics may be prescribed. Treatment with the "cillin" family of antibiotics has been linked with the development of a macular erythematous generalized rash. Mononucleosis is a viral illness that can be caused by CMV, EBV, or adenovirus. The symptoms are generally malaise, fatigue, severe pharyngitis with lymphadonopathy, and fever.

Testing for mononucleosis can be complicated, because the monospot test catches only EBV-related mononucleosis with good sensitivity after 2 weeks of infection. However, the test may not be positive in early infection and is not positive for non-EBV cases. The test stays positive for approximately one year. Alternatively, a blood smear for atypical lymphocytes and evaluation of the differential may hold clues for diagnosis. Treatment of mononucleosis relies mainly on supportive care, fluids, and analgesia. Steroids may be administered if the airway is obstructed; otherwise, no significant benefit is conveyed by their use [23]. Patients in whom mononucleosis is diagnosed can usually be discharged from the ED. They should be instructed to avoid contact sports for 4 to 6 weeks or until they are cleared to resume those activities by their primary care provider because of the risk of splenic rupture.

Peritonsillar abscesses (PTAs) are the most common cause of deep neck infection [24, 25]. PTAs form next to the palatine tonsils and are generally preceded by pharyngitis. The cause is usually polymicrobal, the predominant organisms being GAS, *Staphylococcus aureus* (including methicillin-resistant *Staphylococcus aureus* (MRSA)), and respiratory anaerobes. Patients typically present with a unilateral sore throat, a "hot potato" voice,

and trismus, and they may drool. These patients can have quite an ill appearance and may develop a life-threatening airway obstruction. If trismus is so severe that visualization of the tonsils is limited, CT imaging or examination in an operating room may be required. The typical appearance of a PTA is an extremely swollen, erythematous, fluctuant tonsil. The uvula is deviated to the opposite side. While PTAs are almost always unilateral, bilateral cases may rarely occur and pose a diagnostic challenge.

Imaging is not required to diagnose a PTA, although it may be necessary to differentiate these abscesses from peritonsillar cellulitis and other deep-neck infections. A CT scan with IV contrast is the traditional approach. However, ultrasound imaging is gaining popularity as it offers the advantages of no radiation, immediate results, and real-time guidance for drainage. If the patient has only cellulitis – without abscess formation – antibiotics and supportive care are adequate. If an abscess is present, incision and drainage, either by needle aspiration or with a scalpel, is required. This should be done only by a clinician trained in the procedure. Clindamycin is the preferred antibiotic. For patients with severe infections, vancomycin should be added, particularly if MRSA in the area has a high resistance to clindamycin. Supportive care includes hydration, fever control, analgesia (both systemic and topical), and possibly corticosteroids, with dosing as listed for GAS pharyngitis.

PTA is a potentially life-threatening disease, and it is important to err on the side of transfer to an emergency department. Many patients need to be admitted and need to receive parenteral antibiotics until they are afebrile, tolerate fluids, and show clinical improvement. Reliable patients who have no signs of airway compromise, appear to be otherwise well and have dependable plans for follow-up within 24 hours, may be discharged with a 14-day course of antibiotics.

Retropharyngeal abscess and epiglottitis are two deadly deep-neck infections that must be considered in patients with severe throat pain. Retropharyngeal abscess is much more common in children, but it can occur in adults. Patients are likely to complain of neck stiffness and, typically, appear quite ill. Consider this diagnosis when the severity of the throat pain does not correlate with the physical examination. This condition requires a CT scan for diagnosis, parenteral antibiotics, surgical consultation, and admission. Patients should be transported to the hospital by ambulance.

In the past, epiglottitis was seen more frequently in the very young, but because children are now routinely immunized against *Haemophilus influenza*, older adults have become the primary group with this disease. It is more common among immunocompromised patients, particularly those with HIV infection. Patients with epiglottitis appear fairly sick. They usually sit in a tripod position, have inspiratory stridor, and appear anxious or uncomfortable. Do *not* attempt to manipulate the airway or use invasive measures (including tongue blades) to evaluate the posterior oropharynx. The diagnosis can be made with a lateral neck radiograph, which should be obtained as a portable film because the patient requires constant monitoring for airway obstruction. If this condition is suspected, place the patient in a position of comfort, minimize stimulation, and transport by ambulance to the nearest emergency department as quickly as possible for parenteral antibiotics, ENT consultation, and admission. These patients often need intubation or creation of a surgical airway.

> KEY FACT | **In the past, epiglottitis was seen more frequently in the very young, but older adults have become the primary group with this disease.**

Ear

Ear lacerations have the potential to be extremely disfiguring, especially if they are not repaired correctly. The two most important factors for a successful cosmetic outcome are careful management and coverage of the cartilage and prevention of hematoma formation. The cartilage is avascular and depends on the overlying skin for nutrients and metabolic support. If it is deprived of that support, infection, erosive chondritis, and necrosis can result. This is the process that leads to "cauliflower ear,"

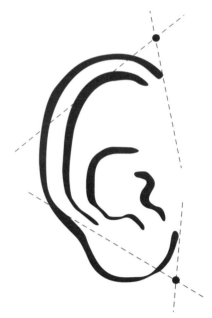

Figure 1.2 Ring block. For the first set of injections, insert the needle superior to the attachment of the ear to the scalp. Direct the needle toward the tragus, aspirate, and inject approximately 2 mL as you pull back. Do *not* remove the needle completely. Redirect posteriorly, along the direction of the helix. Aspirate and inject approximately 2 mL as you pull back. For the second set of injections, insert the needle inferior to the attachment of the earlobe to the scalp. Direct the needle toward the tragus, aspirate, and inject approximately 2 mL as you pull back. Do *not* remove the needle completely. Redirect it posteriorly, along the direction of the helix. Aspirate and inject approximately 2 mL as you pull back.

which may also be caused by blunt trauma. As such a deformity is rarely amenable to reconstruction, prevention is important [27].

> KEY FACT | **The cartilage of the ear is avascular and depends on the overlying skin for nutritional and metabolic support.**

Pitfall | **Failure to cover exposed cartilage and to prevent hematoma formation after acute trauma**

Anesthesia is best provided with either a ring block (Figure 1.2) or a field block. The ring block

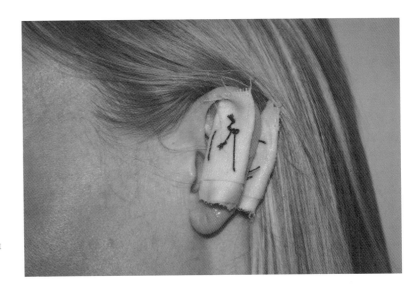

Figure 1.3 Application of a compression dressing will prevent the development of an auricular hematoma.

anesthetizes the entire ear, except for the concha and external auditory canal. The field block, which targets the greater auricular and lesser occipital nerves, anesthetizes the earlobe and lateral helix.

Once the area is numb, appropriate wound repair starts with copious irrigation, just as with any other laceration. Be careful to avoid high pressure, which could dissect the skin away from the cartilage even further. Trim away devitalized cartilage and skin. The cartilage should also be trimmed back if there is insufficient skin to cover it. Up to 5 mm of cartilage can be removed without cosmetic concerns. The next step is approximation of the cartilage. If bringing together the overlying skin accomplishes this goal, this is sufficient. If not, the cartilage should be sutured with 4–0 to 5–0 absorbable sutures. Include the perichondrium in the stitch to prevent tearing the cartilage. Repair the skin with 5–0 to 6–0 non-absorbable sutures, using an interrupted technique [28, 29].

Covering the ear with a bolster or compression dressing is mandatory to prevent development of an auricular hematoma (Figure 1.3).

Follow-up for these patients is critical. The ear must be re-evaluated within 24 hours by an acute care physician or ENT specialist. The dressing must be removed to assess for hematoma and follow-up with ENT should occur within a week.

Lips

Pitfall | **Failure to appropriately repair oral lacerations.**

Lip lacerations are common. When the laceration crosses the vermilion border, proper approximating of the border is critical for producing a satisfactory cosmetic and functional repair. Misalignment of the vermilion border as little as 1 millimeter will result in a cosmetically noticeable scar [28]. The vermilion border should be marked with a pen prior to infiltration of local anesthetic (which can distort local anatomy). An alternative to this approach is the use of a maxillary or mental nerve block instead of local infiltration. Place the first suture through each side of the vermilion, bringing them together. The remainder of the wound can then be closed. If the skin of the face is involved, 5–0 prolene or nylon should be used and can be used for the vermilion border as well; 4–0 chromic gut should be used on the lip. Intraoral lacerations may not always require closure because the mucosa heals very quickly and very well on its own. Large lacerations (greater than 2 cm) and those that interfere with mastication should be closed. An appropriate suture choice is 3–0 chromic gut.

The use of antibiotics in patients with lip lacerations is controversial. Through-and-through lacerations, wounds caused by animal bites, and grossly contaminated wounds are at higher risk for infection, so prophylactic antibiotics are commonly recommended [30]. Both amoxicillin and clindamycin cover oral flora. For all other oral wounds, antibiotics are not necessary. A simple oral antibiotic rinse (e.g. Peridex) is beneficial and can be prescribed if desired [30]. Upon discharge, patients should be instructed to use salt water rinses several times per day, especially after eating, to keep the laceration clean. They can brush their teeth normally. They will need to return for a wound check within 48 hours. The nonabsorbable sutures on the lip should be removed in 5 to 7 days, and the absorbable suture may also be removed at this time if it is still present.

Nose

Pitfall | **Failure to appropriately control epistaxis**

Epistaxis is a common patient presentation in the acute care setting. It occurs more frequently in the winter months because of low humidity levels. Digital trauma, chemical irritants, and infections are common causes. Most cases of epistaxis are self-limited but can be life-threatening with severe bleeds. Bleeds emanate from two primary locations. Anterior bleeds, which are much more common, occur in Kiesselbach's plexus and are often amenable to pressure. Posterior bleeds are most frequently from the sphenopalatine artery and are potentially more serious. The overwhelming majority of patients with epistaxis can be managed by pressure alone and patients should be taught the appropriate location to hold pressure. Pinch the nose with thumb and index finger immediately below the nasal bones. The pressure must be held for a full 5 minutes without interruption. Tilting the head forward is a more effective position, as it maintains patency of the airway and prevents blood from running down the back of the oropharynx.

Pressure works most of the time, but when this technique fails, the key to effective and efficient management is having the proper equipment and setup. Adequate visualization into the nares is mandatory and can be achieved by using good lighting, a nasal speculum, and suction. A topical medication such as oxymetazoline or lidocaine (applied as jelly, nebulized or atomized), should be used for comfort and hemostasis. The application of ice has been taught as a means of inducing hemostasis; it is actually ineffective and uncomfortable [31]. The source of anterior bleeds is typically visible along the nasal septum. Silver nitrate cautery may be used to stop this type of bleeding, but because silver nitrate will not work in a wet field the target area needs to be dried prior to its application. Circumferential cautery around the bleeding site prior to cauterizing the vessel itself is often effective [32]. Never cauterize both sides of the nasal septum, and keep contact to less than 15 seconds to prevent necrosis [33]. Packing may be required if the aforementioned methods fail. If the bleeding source can be visualized, then anterior packing may be sufficient. Numerous commercial devices are available for this purpose. Lubrication, often with lidocaine jelly and oxymetazoline, will make the procedure more comfortable. If hemostasis is achieved with unilateral anterior packing, the patient can be discharged, with ENT follow-up within 24 to 48 hours. Systemic prophylactic antibiotics may not be necessary [34], but most clinicians prescribe anti-staphylococcal antibiotics to prevent toxic shock [35]. All discharged patients should be told to avoid blowing their nose. If posterior or bilateral anterior packing is required, admission to the hospital, typically to an intermediate level of care for airway monitoring, is recommended. Routine laboratory testing is not required for epistaxis. Exceptions, however, include patients with severe bleeding or known bleeding dyscrasias and those who are taking anticoagulation medications. In those cases, a CBC and PT/PTT may be indicated. Patients with renal failure may require a basic metabolic panel (BMP), as uremia compromises platelet function. Hypertension is often thought of as a cause of epistaxis, but in reality arterial hypertension does not cause epistaxis. Hypertension is more likely a result of the stress caused by the bleeding [36]. A blood pressure measurement, taken after the bleeding has been controlled and the patient is calm, will usually be closer to normal.

> KEY FACT | **Arterial hypertension does not cause epistaxis.**

Pearls to improve patient outcomes

• Patients with corneal abrasions, ulcers, and corneal foreign bodies are all treated with antibiotics and should see an ophthalmologist within 24 hours.
• Contact lens wearers with corneal abrasions or patients with corneal ulcers (regardless of contact lens use) require antipseudomonal antibiotic coverage and should be advised to refrain from wearing their contacts until they are cleared to do so by an ophthalmologist.
• Provide systemic corticosteroids to patients with severe throat pain due to GAS pharyngitis in order to hasten symptomatic improvement.
• Consider peritonsillar abscess in patients with a sore throat affecting only one side.
• When patients have throat pain that is out of proportion to the physical findings, consider retropharyngeal abscess and epiglottitis.
• Admit patients with posterior and bilateral anterior packing for control of nosebleeds.

Acknowledgment

This chapter was copyedited by Linda J. Kesselring, MS, ELS, the technical editor/writer in the Department of Emergency Medicine at the University of Maryland School of Medicine.

References

1 Khan FH, Silverberg MA. Corneal abrasion in emergency medicine. Updated on October 25, 2010. Available at emedicine.medscape.com/article/799316-overview. Accessed on February 17, 2011.

2 Jacobs DS. Corneal abrasions and corneal foreign bodies. Updated on September 20, 2010. Available at www.UpToDate.com. Accessed on February 17, 2011.

3 Arbour JD, Brunette I, Boisjoly HM, *et al.* Should we patch corneal erosions? *Arch Ophthalmol* 1997; **115**: 313–317.

4 Blaivas M, Theodoro D, Sierzenski PR. A study of bedside ocular ultrasonography in the emergency department. *Acad Emerg Med* 2002; **9**: 791–799.

5 Sankar PS, Chen TC, Grosskreutz CL, *et al.* Traumatic hyphema. *Int Ophthalmol Clin* 2002; **42**: 57–68.

6 Brandt MT, Haug RH. Traumatic hyphema: a comprehensive review. *J Oral Maxillofac Surg* 2001; **59**: 1462–1470.

7 Walton W, Von Hagen S, Grigorian R, *et al. Management of traumatic hyphema. Surv Ophthalmol* 2002; **47**: 297–334.

8 Snow V, Mottur-Pilson C, Cooper RJ, *et al.* Principles of appropriate antibiotic use for acute pharyngitis in adults. *Ann Intern Med* 2001; **134**: 506–508.

9 Costelloe C, Metcalfe C, Lovering A, *et al.* Effect of antibiotic prescribing in primary care on antimicrobial resistance in individual patients: systematic review and meta-analysis. *BMJ* 2010; **340**: c2096.

10 Del Mar CB, Glasziou PP, Spinks AB. Antibiotics for sore throat. *Cochr Database Syst Rev* 2006 Oct 18; **4**: CD000023.

11 Gerber MA, Shulman ST. Rapid diagnosis of pharyngitis caused by group A streptococci. *Clin Microbiol Rev* 2004; **17**: 571–580.

12 Gieseker KE, Mackenzie T, Roe MH, *et al.* Comparison of two rapid *Streptococcus pyogenes* diagnostic tests with a rigorous culture standard. *Pediatr Infect Dis J* 2002; **21**: 922–927.

13 Kurtz B, Kurtz M, Roe M, *et al.* Importance of inoculum size and sampling effect in rapid antigen detection for diagnosis of *Streptococcus pyogenes* pharyngitis. *J Clin Microbiol* 2000; **38**: 279–281.

14 McIsaac WJ, Kellner JD, Aufricht P *et al.* Empirical validation of guidelines for the management of pharyngitis in children and adults. *JAMA* 2004; **291**: 1587–1595.

15 Humair JP, Revaz SA, Bovier P, *et al.* Management of acute pharyngitis in adults: reliability of rapid streptococcal tests and clinical findings. *Arch Intern Med* 2006; **166**: 640–644.

16 Bisno AL, Gerber MA, Gwaltney JM Jr, *et al.* Practice guidelines for the diagnosis and management of group A streptococcal pharyngitis. Infectious Diseases Society of America. *Clin Infect Dis* 2002; **35**: 113–125.

17 Gerber MA, Baltimore RS, Eaton CB. Prevention of rheumatic fever and diagnosis and treatment of acute Streptococcal pharyngitis: a scientific statement from

the American Heart Association Rheumatic Fever, Endocarditis, and Kawasaki Disease Committee of the Council on Cardiovascular Disease in the Young, the Interdisciplinary Council on Functional Genomics and Translational Biology, and the Interdisciplinary Council on Quality of Care and Outcomes Research: endorsed by the American Academy of Pediatrics. *Circulation* 2009; **119**: 1541–1551.

18 Pichichero ME. Pathogen shifts and changing cure rates for otitis media and tonsillopharyngitis. *Clin Pediatr (Phila)* 2006; **45**: 493–502.

19 Pichichero M, Casey J. Comparison of European and U.S. results for cephalosporin versus penicillin treatment of group A streptococcal tonsillopharyngitis. *Eur J Clin Microbiol Infect Dis* 2006; **25**: 354–364.

20 Korb K, Scherer M, Chenot JF. Steroids as adjuvant therapy for acute pharyngitis in ambulatory patients: a systematic review. *Ann Family Med* 2010; **8**: 58–63.

21 Hayward G, Thompson M, Heneghan C, *et al.* Corticosteroids for pain relief in sore throat: systematic review and meta-analysis. *BMJ* 2009; **339**: b2976.

22 Wing A, Villa-Roel C, Yeh B, *et al.* Effectiveness of corticosteroid treatment in acute pharyngitis: a systematic review of the literature. *Acad Emerg Med* 2010; **17**: 476–483.

23 Candy B, Hotopf M. Steroids for symptom control in infectious mononucleosis. *Cochr Database Syst Rev* 2006; **3**: CD004402.

24 Ungkanont K, Yellon RF, Weissman JL *et al.* Head and neck space infections in infants and children. *Otolaryngol Head Neck Surg* 1995; **112**: 375–382.

25 Schraff S, McGinn JD, Derkay CS. Peritonsillar abscess in children: a 10-year review of diagnosis and management. *Int J Pediatr Otorhinolaryngol* 2001; **57**: 213–218.

26 Levine BJ (ed.). *2011 EMRA Antibiotic Guide.* Emergency Medicine Residents' Association, Irving, Texas, 2010.

27 Ghanem T, Rasamny JK, Park SS. Rethinking auricular trauma. *Laryngoscope* 2005; **115**: 1251–1255.

28 Brown DJ, Jaffe JE, Henson JK. Advanced laceration management. *Emerg Med Clin North Am* 2007; **25**: 83–99.

29 Lammers RL. Methods of wound closure: repair of special structures. In: Roberts JR (ed.), *Clinical Procedures in Emergency Medicine* (5th edn.). Philadelphia: Saunders, 2009.

30 Mark DG, Granquist EJ. Are prophylactic oral antibiotics indicated for the treatment of intraoral wounds? *Ann Emerg Med* 2008; **52**: 368–372.

31 Teymoortash A, Sesterhenn A, Kress R, *et al.* Efficacy of ice packs in the management of epistaxis. *Clin Otolaryngol Allied Sci* 2003; **28**: 545–547.

32 Manes RP. Evaluating and managing the patient with nosebleeds. *Med Clin North Am* 2010; **94**: 903–912.

33 Wurman LH, Sack JG, Flannery JV Jr, *et al.* The management of epistaxis. *Am J Otolaryngol* 1992; **13**:193–209.

34 Biswas D, Mal RK. Are systemic prophylactic antibiotics indicated with anterior nasal packing for spontaneous epistaxis? *Acta Otolaryngol* 2009; **129**: 179–181.

35 Frazee TA, Hauser MS. Nonsurgical management of epistaxis. *J Oral Maxillofac Surg* 2000; **58**: 419–424.

36 Theodosis P, Mouktaroudi M, Papadogiannis D, *et al.* Epistaxis of patients admitted in the emergency department is not indicative of underlying arterial hypertension. *Rhinology* 2009; **47**: 260–263.

CHAPTER 2

Management of Genitourinary Complaints

George Willis[1] and Nadia Eltaki[2]
[1] Department of Emergency Medicine, University of Maryland School of Medicine and Mercy Medical Center, Baltimore, MD, USA
[2] Department of Emergency Medicine, University of Maryland Medical Center, Baltimore, MD, USA

Introduction

Genitourinary complaints are common in most acute care centers. Fortunately, the majority of these complaints are straightforward and do not require much intervention. However, some cases exhibit mild presentations of more serious diseases that require a more thorough workup. The acute care provider must maintain a wide-open differential and refrain from misdiagnosing or mismanaging these more acute disease processes.

Pitfall | Over-reliance on a negative urinalysis to rule out renal colic

Nephrolithiasis is an increasingly encountered medical problem, accounting for nearly 600,000 emergency department visits, 2 million primary outpatient visits, and approximately $2.1 billion in health care-related expenditures in the United States per year [1]. Approximately 3–5% of the population will experience urinary tract stones in their lifetime, with up to 50% of these patients susceptible to recurrence within 10 years [2]. The peak incidence of nephrolithiasis occurs between the ages of 35 and 50. Men remain at the greatest risk, with a male-to-female ratio of approximately 3:1 [2]. Common presenting symptoms include flank pain radiating down into the groin, visible distress, urinary frequency and, sometimes, hematuria.

Prior to the use of CT scans for the diagnosis of kidney stones, intravenous pyelogram (IVP) was the preferred modality of diagnosis. Due to the invasiveness and the associated risks of the procedure, a common practice was using the presence of hematuria on urinalysis to rule in a kidney stone. As a kidney stone passes through the ureter, the lumen becomes irritated and can lead to hematuria as evidenced on the urinalysis. With the advent of unenhanced CT scan as a preferred imaging modality, the use of IVP has become less common. However, some acute care providers continue to use a negative urinalysis for hematuria as a screening tool to rule out renal colic.

Unfortunately, this approach often leads to a misdiagnosis that can place the patient at risk for complications of a kidney stone, such as urinary obstruction, hydronephrosis, renal failure, and renal capsule rupture. Using the urinalysis as a screening tool has been shown in several studies to prove insufficient. Urinalysis looking for the presence of hematuria with at least 10 RBC/mL (which for the study was anything higher than "Trace" on the microscopic analysis) was associated with a sensitivity of 84%, a specificity of 48%, and a negative predictive value of 65% for the detection of a kidney stone [3]. A quarter of patients who had nephrolithiasis on CT scan had no RBCs on a microscopic analysis of the urine [3, 4].

Urgent Care Emergencies: Avoiding the Pitfalls and Improving the Outcomes, First Edition.
Edited by Deepi G. Goyal and Amal Mattu.
© 2012 John Wiley & Sons, Ltd. Published 2012 by John Wiley & Sons, Ltd.

KEY FACT | **In one study, a quarter of patients who had nephrolithiasis on CT scan had no RBC's on urinalysis**

A urinalysis remains useful in the workup of flank pain. It can be used to identify other possible causes of flank pain, such as pyelonephritis. Consequently, there can be a concomitant urinary tract infection associated with a kidney stone. These infections are more difficult to treat and usually require hospitalization, parenteral antibiotics, and possible surgical intervention as inadequate antibiotic penetration occurs due to the obstruction. Immediate urologic consultation is recommended for these patients. Urinalysis also detects hematuria, which still warrants outpatient referral to a urologist if the workup yields no cause for the hematuria.

KEY FACT | **A urinary tract infection associated with a kidney stone is a urologic emergency**

The sensitivity and specificity of CT scan for the detection of kidney stones is 96% and 97% respectively [5]. New technology in the realm of CT scanning has produced faster and more precise scanning machines. The limitations that once delayed a patient's stay in the acute care center have significantly decreased so that the diagnosis is now made or excluded in a relatively short period of time. CT scanning can also detect other significant causes of flank pain, even if hematuria is present. Some of these alternative causes can be found in Box 2.1. Hematuria can be present in a number of these pathologic processes; however, hematuria

Box 2.1 Alternative causes of acute flank pain

- Appendicitis
- Diverticulitis
- Testicular/Ovarian torsion
- Pyelonephritis
- Perinephric hematoma
- Renal capsule rupture
- Abdominal Aortic Aneurysm
- Neoplasm (usually causing obstruction)

can be absent leading to no further workup and significant morbidity if missed. Therefore, CT scan is a valuable modality in the evaluation of any patient presenting with flank pain.

Pitfall | **Failure to add medical expulsive therapy to the outpatient treatment of kidney stones**

The majority of individuals with urolithiasis have small (≤5 mm) stones located in the distal ureter [6]. Studies have shown that the spontaneous passage rates for these types of stones range from 71 to 98% [7]. Barring complications of nephrolithiasis and absolute indications for admission, most patients with kidney stones ≤5 mm can be managed on an outpatient basis. Historically, the focus of outpatient therapy has centered on providing adequate analgesia and urologic referral. In recent years, however, medical expulsive therapy has emerged as a useful, albeit underutilized and under-recognized, adjunct. Medical expulsive therapy refers to the use of medications that relax the ureteral smooth muscle and facilitate stone passage. Agents include non-steroidal anti-inflammatories (NSAIDs), calcium-channel blockers, corticosteroids, and α-adrenergic blockers. Several studies report that patients given these medications have significantly higher rates of spontaneous stone passage, reduced time to stone passage, fewer pain episodes, lower pain scores, and need significantly lower doses of analgesics [7].

Calcium-channel blockers (specifically nifedipine) and α-adrenergic blockers (tamsulosin, terazosin, and doxazosin) are perhaps the best studied. Both α-blockers and calcium-channel blockers have been shown to inhibit the contraction of ureteral smooth muscle that cause ureteral spasms, and pain, while allowing for anterograde stone propagation [6]. In a meta-analysis performed by Hollingsworth *et al.*, patients treated with calcium-channel blockers or α-blockers had a 65% greater likelihood of spontaneous stone passage than patients not given these drugs [7]. Further analysis has shown α-blockers to be superior to calcium-channel blockers in facilitating stone passage [8]. Fewer adverse events have also been noted in patients treated with α-blockers than in those treated with calcium-channel blockers (4% vs. 15.2%) [6].

Although no guidelines exist regarding optimal treatment, the well-documented benefits of medical expulsive therapy indicate that health care practitioners should consider a short course of medical expulsive therapy as a viable adjunct in facilitating urinary stone passage for patients amenable to conservative management. Doing so may shorten the course of the patient's symptoms, but also obviate the need for costly additional care and invasive procedures.

> KEY FACT | **Patients with nephrolithiasis had a 65% greater likelihood of spontaneous stone passage when treated with medical expulsive therapy.**

Pitfall | **Failure to recognize and appropriately treat complicated urinary tract infections**

Urinary tract infections (UTIs) are fairly common occurrences in the acute care center, accounting for almost 8 million outpatient visits each year [9]. Women are most affected because of their shorter urethra and proximity to the vagina and the anus. As a result, one-third of women in the US will experience a UTI by the time they are 25 years old and one-half will experience one by 35 years old [10]. UTI not only afflicts our working population, but also the old and young. In the elderly population, it is the second most common infectious cause for hospital admission and was the highest paid Medicare reimbursement in 1998 [11]. In the pediatric population, the incidence is up to 5% of febrile illnesses presenting to a physician. Overall, this very common disease correlates with high healthcare costs as patients frequently present and are invariably placed on some antibiotic regimen.

Once the diagnosis of a urinary tract infection is established, the acute care provider must differentiate between a simple and a complicated infection. This has nothing to do with the severity of symptomology or with significantly abnormal laboratory values. Rather, it describes a patient population that has either a significant comorbidity or a structural or anatomical abnormality of their urogenital system that predisposes them to an increased risk of worsening and/or significant complications. Complications can include urosepsis, acute renal insufficiency, and perinephric abscess. A list of these risk factors is given in Box 2.2. Any patient with these risk factors who is diagnosed with a urinary tract infection needs to be managed as if they have a complicated UTI.

Diabetes mellitus deserves special mention because diabetics are at the highest risk for complications surrounding inadequately treated urinary tract infections. Glucosuria predisposes diabetics to asymptomatic bacteriuria, which usually leads to ascension up the urinary tract leading to a UTI. Because of decreased renal perfusion and decreased immune response, infections with atypical pathogens such as Pseudomonas and fungi can occur and inadequate antimicrobial coverage often results in serious complications. Perinephric abscesses and emphysematous pyelonephritis are complications seen almost exclusively in diabetics and the latter carries a mortality of 25% with likely loss of the affected kidney [12].

> KEY FACT | **Emphysematous pyelonephritis is a complication almost exclusively found in diabetics and carries a mortality of 25%.**

Complicated urinary tract infections require longer regimens of antimicrobial therapy that will

---

Box 2.2 Risk factors for complicated UTI

- Diabetes mellitus
- Male gender
- Children
- Elderly
- Recent hospitalization
- Indwelling catheters
- GU surgery (i.e. nephrostomy, stents)
- Renal insufficiency
- Vesicoureteral reflux
- Urethral valves
- Pregnancy
- Immunocompromised
- Concomitant nephrolithiasis

> **Box 2.3** Treatment regimens for complicated UTI
>
> Outpatient:
>
> - Ciprofloxacin 500 mg bid or Levofloxacin 750 mg once daily
> - Third generation cephalosporin such as ceftibuten, cefdinir, or cefpodoxime
>
> Inpatient:
>
> - Ciprofloxacin 400 mg IV bid or levofloxacin 750 mg IV once daily
> - Third generation cephalosporin such as ceftriaxone, ceftazidime, or cefotaxime
> - Imipenem/Cilastin
> - Piperacillin/Tazobactam

perfuse the urinary tract as well as the parenchyma of the organs involved. The approach to treatment of complicated UTI is to start a broad-spectrum antibiotic after obtaining a urine culture. Treatment regimens can be found in Box 2.3. Fluoroquinolones have been first-line treatment because they maintain heavy concentration in the urine and renal parenchyma. Unless contraindicated (i.e. pregnancy, pediatrics), it is recommended to start with a fluoroquinolone, follow up with the culture results, and adjust therapy accordingly. Disposition is dependent on the patient's presentation, but requires a low threshold to hospitalize these patients for at least a day of parenteral antibiotics. If they are discharged home, they should have very close follow-up (i.e. within 48 hours) to evaluate response to therapy and to amend therapy based on culture results.

Pitfall | Failure to accurately diagnose and manage acute scrotal pain

Acute scrotal pain is an infrequent complaint in the acute care setting. However, a patient who presents with this complaint should have immediate evaluation by the acute care provider to determine the possible causes. Studies have shown that it is difficult to differentiate testicular torsion from torsion of the appendix testis and epididymitis/orchitis based on presenting symptoms and historical features alone [13].

Testicular torsion is one of the most common surgical emergencies occurring in males with an annual incidence of 1 in 4,000 among patients younger than 25 years of age, with a bimodal distribution, the largest peak occurring around puberty (accounting for 65% of all torsions) and another smaller peak in the first year of life [14, 15]. A delay in diagnosis not only risks the viability of the affected testis, but may also cause auto-immune destruction of the uninvolved testes, leading to bilateral testicular damage and reduced fertility [16]. Epididymitis is the fifth most common urologic diagnosis in men between the ages of 18 and 50, with the majority of cases occurring between 20 and 39 years [17]. Among sexually active men younger than 35 years, acute epididymitis is most frequently caused by sexually transmitted organisms, specifically *Chlamydia trachomatis* and *Neisseria gonorrhoeae*. In contrast, the most common pathogens isolated in infectious epididymitis in men > 35 years are coliform bacteria, with *Escherichia coli* accounting for the majority of cases [18, 19].

Differentiating between these two etiologies for acute scrotal pain is a diagnostic dilemma for the acute care provider. While some studies suggest that patients with testicular torsion tend to present earlier than other diagnoses, this historical element should not be used to distinguish between these entities alone. Furthermore, the classic pattern of acute-onset unilateral testicular pain may not be present in all cases. In a retrospective review of patients with testicular torsion, 89% of patients presented with this symptom. The investigators also found associated groin, abdominal, or thigh pain in 34% of these patients, indicating that alternative areas of pain may represent the earliest or predominant symptom in testicular torsion [14].

The physical examination findings in patients who present with acute scrotal pain may also be misleading. Specifically, the absence of the cremasteric reflex (which is considered the most sensitive physical examination finding in testicular torsion) may be unreliable. In a study of 225 healthy boys, investigators noted the cremasteric reflex was present in all boys older than 30 months but in less than half of those younger than 30 months [20]. Likewise, Prehn's sign, commonly used to differentiate torsion from epididymitis by relief of pain when the testicle inflamed by epididymitis is elevated, is not specific [21]. Other classic physical examination findings that suggest testicular torsion, including a higher lie of the affected testis, horizontal lie of the contralateral testis, and displacement of the epididymis from its usual posterior position may not be present, and the absence of any one or more of these findings should not be used to rule out the diagnosis of torsion.

> KEY FACT | **In healthy children less than 30 months old, less than half had a cremasteric reflex, making it an unreliable physical exam finding when evaluating for torsion.**

Because of these diagnostic dilemmas and the potentially disastrous outcome in delay of diagnosis, it is critical for the acute care provider to consider testicular torsion in all cases of acute scrotal pain. When the diagnosis of testicular torsion is questionable, the provider must obtain Doppler ultrasonography and/or urologic consultation expeditiously. Only after the diagnosis of torsion has been excluded should other diagnoses be considered.

If epididymitis is the diagnosis, the patient must be managed appropriately. Only half of patients 18–35 years with a diagnosis of epididymitis receive appropriate treatment [22, 23]. Per CDC recommendations, empiric therapy for epididymitis is indicated before laboratory results are available and should be guided by the patient's age and sexual history. Testing for *N. gonorrhoeae* and *C. trachomatis* should be performed in sexually active patients <35 years using the diagnostic modality readily available to the clinician (i.e. culture, nucleic acid hybridization test, or nucleic acid amplification test). Treatment regimens can be found in Box 2.4. Adjunctive treatment modalities, including bed rest, scrotal elevation, and analgesics, are also recommended until fever and inflammation have subsided [24, 25]. Of equal importance to choosing the appropriate antibiotic regimen is thorough patient education. Patients who have acute epididymitis that is suspected or confirmed to be caused by *N. gonorrhoeae* or *C. trachomatis* should be instructed to refer recent sexual partners

> **Box 2.4** Treatment regimens for acute epididymitis
>
> For acute epididymitis most likely caused by gonococcal or chlamydial infection:
> - ceftriaxone 250 mg IM in a single dose
>
>   PLUS
> - doxycycline 100 mg orally twice a day for 10 days
>
> For acute epididymitis most likely caused by enteric organisms or with negative confirmatory gonococcal testing:
> - ofloxacin 300 mg orally twice a day for 10 days
>
>   OR
> - levofloxacin 500 mg orally once daily for 10 days

(within 60 days) for evaluation and treatment. In addition, they should be instructed to abstain from sexual intercourse until they and their partners have been adequately treated [24].

Pitfall | **Failure to suspect pregnancy**

Every woman of childbearing age should be presumed pregnant until proven otherwise. Multiple studies have shown that historical and physical exam features are inconsistent and unreliable in determining the possibility of pregnancy. Despite recording various historical variables – including the date of the patient's last menstrual period, whether the patient's menstrual period was on time, birth control usage, and whether the patient suspected she was pregnant – one study showed that there was still a 10% chance of pregnancy being overlooked [26]. Furthermore, women may not associate certain symptoms with early pregnancy. One study showed that among fertile patients who presented to the emergency department for any reason, the prevalence of unrecognized pregnancy (defined as a "pregnancy not definitely known to exist") in those with abdominal pain or pelvic complaints was found to be 13% [27]. Conversely, the absence of early symptoms of pregnancy, such as morning sickness, does not rule out pregnancy [28].

Although patients may report results based on home pregnancy testing, acute care providers should maintain a fair amount of skepticism. In a study by Doshi, the accuracy of three in-home pregnancy tests was found to be only 77% [29]. These findings highlight that the accuracy of home pregnancy tests relies on several factors, including the ability of patients to carefully follow the test kit instructions, the timing of testing (i.e. number of days beyond the missed menstrual period), and the ease with which test results can be interpreted.

Given the poor reliability of the patient's history in determining pregnancy status, and the potential disastrous outcomes of missing the diagnoses of pregnancy (i.e. prescribing teratogenic studies and therapies), it is recommended that laboratory testing (urine or serum HCG) be performed to determine the diagnoses of pregnancy.

Pitfall | **Failure to treat asymptomatic bacteriuria in pregnancy**

Asymptomatic bacteriuria is an infection of the genitourinary system where the patient does not experience any symptoms. In the majority of patients, it is an incidental finding on a urinalysis that is usually being ordered for another reason. Because of the close proximity of the urethra to the genital tract in women and the short length of the urethra, the prevalence of asymptomatic bacteriuria in the young adult population is fairly common, somewhere between 2 and 10% [30] and more prevalent in populations from lower socioeconomic status. Failure to treat asymptomatic bacteriuria in most patient populations will typically result in no adverse events. In these cases, the infection will most commonly be cleaned out by the body's immune response or, rarely, will progress to a symptomatic infection resulting in the patient seeking medical attention.

However, the pregnant population deserves special attention when it comes to asymptomatic bacteriuria. Hormone changes cause the ureter and the bladder to relax causing stagnation of urinary flow through the urinary tract. Ureteral compression and obstruction by the gravid uterus causes further slowing of urinary flow down the ureters. Glucose in the urine serves as a medium for bacterial growth. These pregnancy-associated physiologic changes place the patient at risk for ascension of the bacteria up the urinary tract causing worsening infection. Thirty percent of preg-

nant patients who have untreated asymptomatic bacteriuria go on to develop pyelonephritis, which places them at risk for kidney failure, sepsis, and ARDS [31].

There are also risks for the fetus. Pregnancies associated with untreated asymptomatic bacteriuria are also at increased risk of preterm labor and delivery as well as low birth weight babies. Patients without asymptomatic bacteriuria were half as likely to experience preterm delivery and two-thirds as likely to deliver a low-birth weight infant [30–32]. For this reason, prenatal clinics screen for asymptomatic bacteriuria as primary prevention for the complications. However, patients of lower socioeconomic status are more likely to delay or never establish prenatal care and will often present to acute care centers for any complaints that may occur during the pregnancy. Fortunately, a common practice in most acute care centers is to confirm a pregnancy with a urine pregnancy test. It is recommended that the acute care provider also check a urinalysis in combination with the pregnancy test to screen for asymptomatic bacteriuria.

> KEY FACT | **30% of pregnant patients with untreated asymptomatic bacteriuria go on to develop pyelonephritis.**

Contrary to the common practice in nonpregnant patients, the current recommendations are to treat asymptomatic bacteriuria with antibiotics in pregnant patients. Treatment has been shown to decrease the risk of pyelonephritis by 80% and the risk of low-birth weight infants by 15% [31]. There has been an increase in *E. coli* resistant to ampicillin, making the penicillins obsolete. Cephalosporins and nitrofurantoin are the most commonly used antibiotics for the treatment of asymptomatic bacteriuria and are equally effective.

> KEY FACT | **Treating asymptomatic bacteriuria in pregnancy decreases the risk of pyelonephritis by 80% and the risk of low-birth weight infants by 15%.**

Pitfall | **Failure to consider ovarian torsion in females who present with acute lower abdominal pain**

Ovarian torsion is a frequently taught, yet highly under-recognized cause of acute abdominal pain. It is the fifth most common gynecological emergency, accounting for 2.7% of acute gynecologic complaints [33, 34]. Early diagnosis and treatment is essential in order to salvage the affected ovary. Unfortunately, delay in diagnosis is more common, leading to a reported ovarian salvage rate of less than 10% [33].

> KEY FACT | **Due to delay in diagnosis of ovarian torsion, the rate of ovarian salvage once the diagnosis is made is less than 10%.**

The challenges to establishing an early diagnosis of ovarian torsion are multifactorial. Classically, patients with ovarian torsion present with abrupt onset, colicky, unilateral lower abdominal pain that radiates to the flank or groin and progressively worsens over several hours. In one study, however, this "classic" presentation was only found in 44% of patients with confirmed ovarian torsion [35].

> KEY FACT | **The "classic" presentation for ovarian torsion was found in only 44% of patients with confirmed ovarian torsion.**

Furthermore, the differential diagnosis for patients presenting with such complaints is broad and may include other emergency causes such as ectopic pregnancy, pelvic inflammatory disease, appendicitis, diverticulitis, ovarian cyst, and renal colic [33]. The frequent occurrence of these particular diseases may lead the acute care provider to overlook the less common diagnosis of ovarian torsion as the cause of the patient's acute abdominal pain. In fact, in a retrospective analysis of patients with surgically confirmed ovarian torsion, the diagnosis of ovarian torsion was considered in the admitting differential in only 47% of cases [35]. Moreover, physical exam findings are highly variable and may be misleading. In a study by Houry et al, one third of patients with surgically confirmed ovarian torsion had only mild tenderness on abdominal examination, while 29% had no tenderness on pelvic examination [35]. The same study also showed that almost half of these patients (47%)

had a palpable mass on pelvic examination, but more than half (53%) had a known diagnosis of ovarian cyst or mass [35]. This finding reflects the ease with which a known ovarian cyst or mass may cloud the new diagnosis of ovarian torsion and lead the provider to dismiss the patient's acute findings as a manifestation of her chronic pathology.

Though the diagnosis of ovarian torsion may be elusive based on history and physical examination alone, it is essential for the health care practitioner to consider it in the differential diagnosis of all female patients who present with acute lower abdominal pain. In cases when the diagnosis is likely, prompt sonographic evaluation and gynecologic consultation should be pursued.

Pitfall | **Failure to diagnose and treat pelvic inflammatory disease due to lack of symptoms**

Pelvic inflammatory disease (PID) is an infection of the upper genital tract in women. Most commonly caused by sexually transmitted infections (STI), such as *Neisseria gonorrhoeae* and *Chlamydia trachomatis*, PID is most prevalent in the young and sexually active population. The prevalence has been declining since the 1980s due to a heightened awareness in the general population and the increase in free STI clinics [36]. However, the rate of misdiagnosis remains high leading to a number of complications including tubo-ovarian abscess, increased risk of ectopic pregnancy, and infertility.

The diagnosis of PID is very difficult due to variable presentation ranging from mild pelvic pain to peritonitis. The so-called "classic presentation" for PID of pelvic pain, vaginal discharge, and fever is frequently not found. There is not a single finding in the history, physical examination, or laboratory studies that is sensitive or specific for the diagnosis of PID. Even in the hands of experts, the history and physical examination were found to have a positive predictive value of only 65–90% [36, 37]. Furthermore, the presentation can often mimic other disease processes that may lead the acute care practitioner to pursue other diagnoses, such as appendicitis or a urinary tract infection.

KEY FACT | **The history and physical has a positive predictive value of 65–90% for the clinical diagnosis of PID.**

In 2010, the CDC recognized the difficulty in making the diagnosis of PID. Consequently, they simplified the diagnostic criteria in an attempt to lower the threshold to diagnose and treat. The diagnostic criteria can be found in Box 2.5.

In addition to these diagnostic criteria, the acute care provider must also consider patient risk factors. Patients who are considered high-risk patients are found in Box 2.6. Patients who are considered high risk who complain of abdominal or pelvic pain without an alternative etiology for their pain should be treated empirically for PID. Obtain laboratory studies as well, including swabs from the cervix for culture. However, because of the processing time of cervical cultures, the diagnosis should be made and antimicrobial therapy started prior to the results of the cultures returning.

Treatment consists of antimicrobials directed against both *N. gonorrhoeae* and *C. trachomatis* as the clinical spectrum of either infection by these pathogens is similar. Treatment regimens can be found in Box 2.7. Cure with these CDC-recommended regimens have been found to be more than 90% effective; treatment failure is usually due to noncompliance or presence of a TOA [36]. Hospitalization for parenteral antimicrobial administration is necessary in certain circumstances such as pregnancy or inability to tolerate oral medications. However, several studies have shown that treatment with oral and parenteral medications are equally as effective.

Box 2.5 Diagnostic criteria for pelvic inflammatory disease [37]

Minimum criteria
Presence of one or more of the following on pelvic examination:
- cervical motion tenderness
- adnexal tenderness
- uterine tenderness.

Presence of the following in addition to the minimum criteria enhances the specificity for the diagnosis:
- fever
- infection with *C. trachomatis* or *N. gonorrhoeae*
- elevated ESR and/or CRP
- vaginal or cervical mucopurulent discharge.

Box 2.6 Risk factors for PID

- Younger age of onset of sexual activity
- Multiple sexual partners
- Low socioeconomic status
- Prior history of sexually transmitted infections
- Intercourse without barrier contraception
- Intercourse during menses

Box 2.7 CDC recommended treatment regimen for PID

Outpatient:
- ceftriaxone 250 mg IM × 1 dose
  PLUS
- doxycycline 100 mg PO bid for 14 days
  +/−
- metronidazole 500 mg PO bid for 14 days

  OR
- cefoxitin 2 g IM × 1 dose and probenecid 1 g PO × 1 dose
  PLUS
- doxycycline 100 mg PO bid for 14 days
  +/−
- metronidazole 500 mg PO bid for 14 days

  OR
- other parenteral third-generation cephalosporin (e.g. ceftizoxime or cefotaxime)
  PLUS
- doxycycline 100 mg PO bid for 14 days
  +/−
- metronidazole 500 mg PO bid for 14 days

Inpatient:
- cefotetan 2 g intravenously (IV) every 12 h

  OR
- cefoxitin 2 g IV every 6 h
  PLUS
- doxycycline 100 mg orally or IV every 12 h

Pearls for improving patient outcomes

- A urinalysis is inadequate when used as a screening tool for ruling in or out nephrolithiasis.
- Remember to include expulsive therapy to increase the success rate of nephrolithiasis passage.
- Always consider whether a urinary tract infection is complicated and treat appropriately and for an adequate amount of time.
- A female of child-bearing age is pregnant until proven otherwise with sufficient laboratory testing.
- Always screen for and treat asymptomatic bacteriuria in any pregnant patient.
- Rule out the diagnosis of testicular torsion in any patient with acute scrotal pain.
- Patients with epididymitis should be tested and treated for *N. gonorrhoeae* and *C. trachomatis* infections, especially in the sexually active population.
- Consider the diagnosis of PID in any patient who presents with acute pelvic pain with no other explanation and treat empirically.

References

1 Pearle MS, Calhoun EA, Curhan GC, *et al*. Urologic disease in America project: urolithiasis. *J Urol* 2005; **173**: 848–857.

2 Menon M, Parulkar BG, Drach GW. Urinary lithiasis: etiology, diagnosis, and medical management. In: Walsh PC, *et al*. (eds.), *Campbell's Urology* (7th edn.). WB Saunders: Philadelphia, 1998: 2661–2705.

3 Luchs JS, Katz DS, *et al*. Utility of hematuria testing in patients with suspected renal colic: correlation with unenhanced helical CT results. *Urology* 2002; **59**: 839–842.

4 Bove P, Kaplan D, *et al*. Reexamining the value of hematuria testing in patients with acute flank pain. *J Urol* 1999; **162**: 685–687.

5 Smith RC, Verga M, *et al*. Diagnosis of acute flank pain: value of unenhanced helical CT. *AJR* 1996; **166**: 97–101.

6 Singh A, Alter HJ, Littlepage A. A systematic review of medical therapy to facilitate passage of ureteral calculi. *Ann Emerg Med* 2007; **50**: 552–563.

7 Hollingsworth JM, Rogers MA, Kaufman SR, *et al*. Medical therapy to facilitate urinary stone passage: a meta-analysis. *Lancet* 2006; **368**: 1171–1179.

8 Preminger GM, Tiselius HG, Assimos DG, *et al*. 2007 Guideline for the Management of Ureteral Calculi. *Eur Urol* 2007; **52**: 1610–1631.

9 Stamm WE, Hooton TM. Management of urinary tract infections in adults. *N Engl J Med* 1993; **329**(18): 1328–1334.

10 Foxman B, Barlow R, D'Arcy H, *et al*. Urinary tract infection: self-reported incidence and associated costs. *Ann Epidemiol* 2000; **10**: 509–15.

11 Litwin MS, Saigal CS, Beerbohm EM. The burden of urologic diseases in America. *J Urol* 2005; **173**: 1605–1606.

12 Falagas ME, Alexiou VG, Giannopoulou KP, *et al*. Risk factors for mortality in patients with emphysematous pyelonephritis: a meta-analysis. *J Urol* 2007; **178**(3): 880–885.

13 Ringdahl E, Teague L. Testicular torsion. *Am Fam Phys* 2006; **74**: 1739–1743.

14 Anderson J, Williamson R. Testicular torsion in Bristol: a 25 year review. *Br J Surg* 1988; **294**: 825.

15 Melekos M, Asbach H, Markou S. Etiology of the acute scrotum with regard to age distribution. *J Urol* 1998; **139**: 1023–1025.

16 Rabinowitz R, Nagler H, Kogan S, *et al*. Experimental aspects of testicular torsion. *Dialog Paediat Urol* 1985; **8**: 1–8.

17 Collins MM, Stafford RS, O'Leary MP, *et al*. How common is prostatitis? A national survey of physician visits. *J Urol* 1998; **159**: 1224–1228.

18 Tracy CR, Steers WD, Costabile RA. Diagnosis and management of epididymitis. *Urol Clin North Am* 2008; **35**: 101–108.

19 Luzzi GA, O'Brien TS. Acute epididymitis. *BJU Int* 2001; **87**: 747–755.

20 Caesar RE, Kaplan GW. The incidence of the cremasteric reflex in normal boys. *J Urol* 1994; **102**: 779–780.

21 Haynes BE, Bessen HA, Haynes VE. The diagnosis of testicular torsion. *JAMA* 1983; **249**: 2522–2527.

22 Tracy CR, Costabile RA. The evaluation and treatment of acute epididymitis in a large university based population: are CDC guidelines being followed? *World J Urol* 2009; **27**: 259–263.

23 Drury NE, Dyer JP, Breitenfeldt N, *et al*. Management of acute epididymitis: are European guidelines being followed? *Eur Urol* 2004; **46**: 522–525.

24 Workowsk KA, Berman, SM. Sexually transmitted diseases treatment guidelines, 2006. Center for Disease Control and Prevention. *MMWR* 2006; **55**: 1–94.

25 Center for Disease Control and Prevention. Updated recommended treatment regimens for gonococcal infections and associated conditions – United States, April 2007. http://www.cdc.gov/std/treatment/2006/GonUpdateApril2007.pdf

26 Ramoska E. Reliability of patient history in determining the possibility of pregnancy. *Ann Emerg Med* 1989; **18**: 48–50.

27 Stengel CL, Seaberg DC, Macleod BA. Pregnancy in the emergency department: risk factors and prevalence among women. *Ann Emerg Med* 1994; **24**: 697–700.

28 Bastian LA, Piscitelli JT. Is this patient pregnant? Can you reliably rule in or out early pregnancy by clinical examination? *JAMA* 1997; **278**: 586–591.

29 Doshi ML. Accuracy of consumer-performed in-home tests for early pregnancy detection. *Am J Public Health* 1986; **76**: 512–514.

30 Sheiner E, Mazor-Drey E, Levy A. Asymptomatic bacteriuria during pregnancy. *J Mat-Fetal Neonat Med* 2009; **22**(5): 423–427.

31 Millar L, Cox S. Urinary tract infections complicating pregnancy. *Infect Dis Clin North Am* 1997; **11**: 13–26.

32 Romero R, Oyarzun E, Mazor M, *et al* Meta-analysis of the relationship between asymptomatic bacteriuria and preterm delivery/low birth weight. *Obstet Gynecol* 1989; **73**: 576–582.

33 Hibbard LT. Adnexal torsion. *Am J Obstet Gynecol* 1985; **152**: 456–461.

34 Burnett LS. Gynecologic causes of the acute abdomen. *Surg Clin North Am* 1988; **68**: 385–398.

35 Houry D, Abbott JT. Ovarian torsion: a fifteen-year review. *Ann Emerg Med* 2001; **38**: 156–159.

36 Lareau SM, Beigi RH. Pelvic inflammatory disease and tubo-ovarian abscess. *Infect Dis Clin North Am* 2008; **22**: 693–708.

37 Workowski K, Berman S. Sexually Transmitted Diseases Treatment Guidelines, 2010. *MMWR* 2010; **59**: 1–116.

CHAPTER 3

Orthopedic Pitfalls of the Upper Extremity

Brooks M. Walsh[1] and Reinier van Tonder[2]

[1] Department of Emergency Medicine, Bridgeport Hospital, Yale New Haven Health System, Bridgeport, CT, USA

[2] Department of Emergency Medicine, Kaiser Permanente, San Diego Medical Center, San Diego, CA, USA

Introduction

The upper extremities are subject to a variety of traumatic and infectious insults. Estimates of the incidence of these disorders range widely, but approximately a third of the general population will have an upper extremity musculoskeletal disorder in their lifetime [1]. Many of these patients will receive their initial evaluation in the urgent care setting. Although most complaints will have a straightforward presentation, the acute care provider must be skilled in the evaluation of a number of important clinical issues in order to avoid pitfalls.

Pitfall | Failure to diagnose a posterior shoulder dislocation

The majority of shoulder dislocations are anterior and are suggested by physical examination findings as well as standard radiographs. However, approximately 3%, present as a posterior dislocation. The relative rarity of this disorder accounts in part for the high initial misdiagnosis rate with as many as 79% missed on the initial presentation. Diagnosis can also be difficult due to concomitant fractures, typically of the proximal humerus, that obscure the acute presentation. A subacute presentation may be confused with adhesive capsulitis [2]. Perhaps the most salient reason for missing the diagnosis is

not considering the diagnosis, and thus not ordering the appropriate imaging to exclude it.

There are a number of soft-tissue and osseous stabilizers of the shoulder that prevent posterior dislocation, but certain mechanisms are more likely to overcome these. The shoulder is stabilized, in part, by sets of muscles that act as external and internal rotators of the humerus. The external rotators are much weaker than the internal ones, and thus a strong contraction of both sets, such as may happen in an electrical injury or a generalized tonic–clonic seizure, will preferentially pull the humeral head out of its position. A posterior dislocation may also be caused by a fall onto a shoulder held in forward flexion, adducted, and in internal rotation [3, 4].

A missed opportunity to diagnose this entity can result in degenerative changes in the joint, avascular necrosis, and disability [5]. Despite the infrequent presentation, a few simple elements of the physical examination can either suggest or rule out the diagnosis.

Inspection of the shoulder may show a prominent coracoid process and an anterior "void." The humeral head may be visualized or palpable posteriorly [5]. These findings may be subtle, however, and further examination of the passive and active range of motion of the shoulder is warranted. The affected arm will, as a rule, be held in an adducted, internally rotated position. The patient will be

Urgent Care Emergencies: Avoiding the Pitfalls and Improving the Outcomes, First Edition.
Edited by Deepi G. Goyal and Amal Mattu.
© 2012 John Wiley & Sons, Ltd. Published 2012 by John Wiley & Sons, Ltd.

unable to externally rotate the humerus, or to supinate the ipsilateral forearm, to any significant degree, either actively or passively [2, 3].

> KEY FACT | **The inability to externally rotate the humerus or to supinate the palm suggests a posterior dislocation.**

Shoulder radiographs are commonly ordered for the evaluation of the shoulder following trauma, and typically comprise anteroposterior (AP) and lateral views. There are a number of subtle signs on the AP view that may indicate a posterior dislocation. A coincident proximal humerus fracture will be found in about half of these dislocations, but the finding of a dramatic fracture should not distract the acute care provider from fully examining the radiograph [3]. The humerus may appear internally rotated, with disappearance of the greater tuberosity as it moves from the lateral to an anterior position. The resulting symmetric appearance of the humeral head and tapering shaft have suggested the colloquial "light bulb" and "ice-cream cone" signs. The normal oval area of overlap between the humeral head and the glenoid may be widened, or show diminished or uneven overlap (see Figure 3.1). If an impression fracture of the humeral head has formed, it may be visible as a parallel line, just lateral to the medial border of the humerus (the "trough" sign). Unfortunately, all these signs may be absent or difficult to discern. The trough sign may be found in only 64% of AP films, while the "light bulb" in only 28% [6]. An isolated fracture of the lesser tuberosity should lead one to suspect posterior dislocation of the shoulder until proven otherwise [7].

As the AP and thoracic lateral views are insensitive for detecting a posterior dislocation, additional views are required. The scapular "Y-view" may be helpful, but can be unreliable due to patient positioning issues or subtle presentations. The axillary view, however, reliably determines the position of the humeral head and is the best for discerning posterior dislocation. Unlike the scapular "Y-view," unfortunately, the shoulder must be moved to obtain the image, with 15–20 degrees of abduction required.

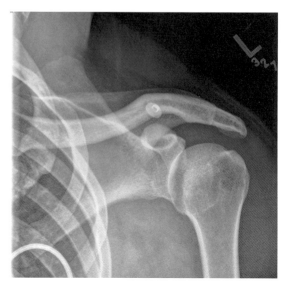

Figure 3.1 Posterior shoulder dislocation. AP view with posterior shoulder dislocation.

If a posterior dislocation is diagnosed, orthopedic referral is required and transfer to the emergency room is warranted.

> KEY FACT | **The axillary view should be ordered for all patients with potential shoulder injuries or humeral injuries as it is the most sensitive means of identifying posterior shoulder dislocation.**

Pitfall | Failure to consider septic bursitis in the patient with a swollen elbow

Bursae are small, fluid-filled sacs that serve to facilitate motion between layers of tissue, e.g. between skin and bone. Some of these bursae are deep, such as the iliopsoas bursa, and others are superficial. Inflammation of these bursae can result from various infectious and noninfectious etiologies. Bursitis most commonly affects the superficial prepatellar and olecranon bursae [8]. Non-infectious bursitis can be the result of acute or chronic trauma, a crystal arthropathy, or rheumatoid arthritis. These factors can also predispose the bursae to subsequent infection, however [8].

Infectious, or septic, bursitis is typically triggered by a direct percutaneous mechanism, as would happen with a traumatic injury, or by spread from an overlying cellulitis. While there can be a coincident septic arthritis, a joint space infection usually results from hematogenous seeding, whereas bacteremia is very unusual in septic bursitis [8, 9].

The majority of cases of septic bursitis are due to *Staphylococcus aureus* [10]. Unlike septic arthritis, the risk of methicillin-resistant *S. aureus* (MRSA) in septic bursitis is not well elucidated. Case reports show a documented MRSA bursitis in only a few instances, involving either severe immunosuppression [11] or instrumentation [12].

> KEY FACT | **Septic bursitis, unlike septic arthritis, does not significantly affect the range of motion.**

Septic olecranon bursitis typically presents as a tender, swollen, and erythematous elbow. The swelling is described as locally edematous, with the maximum tenderness centered on the bursa [8]. Unlike septic arthritis, the active range of motion should not be significantly affected. Elements of the history and physical examination that differentiate septic bursitis from noninfectious causes are a shorter duration of symptoms, a greater degree of pain and tenderness, and increased erythema [13–16]. These differences are of uncertain value for definitive diagnosis. A fever is found in about half of the septic cases, but none of the nonseptic cases [14, 16, 10]. Perhaps more useful is the finding that the skin over a septic bursitis is consistently judged to be warmer than the contralateral elbow [13, 14], and so a "cold" elbow provides good support for a nonseptic etiology.

Studies of the blood for sedimentation rate and white blood count are of marginal utility, as the values for septic and nonseptic bursitis overlap to a great degree [8, 10, 17].

The gold standard for diagnosis of a septic bursitis is a culture of the bursal fluid. Most authorities recommend aspiration of the bursa to establish if there is any suspicion in the diagnosis.

A diagnostic aspiration should be performed with the elbow in flexion at 90 degrees; the increased intrabursal pressure will aid in complete drainage [18]. Employ an 18-g needle with a 20-ml syringe.

Use a sterile technique, and clean the area with chlorhexidine or an equivalent antiseptic cleanser. The site of needle entry must be free of signs of infection, such as cellulitis. The needle is directed parallel to the forearm along the lateral aspect, avoiding the ulnar nerve [38]. After an anesthetic wheal is placed, the aspiration is performed with the aim of draining the bursa; "milking" of the sac may be required. A bandage and compressive dressing should be applied after the procedure [18].

Bursal fluid should be analyzed for cell count, Gram stain, glucose, culture, and, if gout is suspected, crystals. It is important to keep in mind, however, that septic fluid may only be moderately turbid, while a seemingly purulent aspirate may have a noninfectious cause; e.g. gout. Similarly, the initial studies may not be diagnostic. There is no cutoff value for the cell count that defines septic bursitis [10, 13, 15].

Despite the support for diagnostic aspiration, there are concerns that complications, such as seeding of the bursa or fistulization of the tract, may complicate treatment. Although there is little support in the literature to support the practice, many practitioners elect to defer diagnostic aspiration on the initial visit, and employ empiric antibiotics. Regardless of the diagnostic approach, it is mandatory that re-evaluation be arranged for 48–72 hours later.

> KEY FACT | **All patients with a possible septic bursitis require re-evaluation within 48–72 hours.**

Recommendations for treatment generally involve 2–3 weeks of a beta-lactamase antibiotic. A suggested regimen is dicloxacillin 500 mg four times daily [19]. A number of references advise coverage for MRSA in patients with severe disease, past history of MRSA infection, or risk factors for MRSA colonization. Outpatient treatment may be appropriate for most mild and moderate cases, but early follow-up is required in all cases to assure adequate therapy and assessment for repeated drainage.

Pitfall | **Failure to recognize a potential scaphoid injury**

The scaphoid bone of the wrist, named for its resemblance to a boat with rounded prow and stern, occupies both a precarious location anatomically, as well as a prominent placement in the list in the pitfalls. Although the majority of carpal bone fractures are of the scaphoid, diagnosis can be hampered by a number of difficulties in physical evaluation and diagnostic imaging, as well as the potential for significant costs in both over- and under-treatment.

The scaphoid bone bridges both the proximal and distal rows of carpal bones. It acts to block wrist extension, and abuts the distal radius. These anatomic factors make the scaphoid vulnerable in a fall onto an outstretched hand (FOOSH) [20]. Furthermore, the blood supply to this bone is tenuous. Two branches off of the radial artery enter the bone distally, and so the proximal pole is supplied only by a retrograde interosseous blood flow. This predisposes fractures of the proximal pole to avascular necrosis and resorption [20].

Any patient with a history of trauma to a distal upper extremity should receive a full musculoskeletal and neurovascular examination. This should include an evaluation for scaphoid bone injury, especially if there is a history of a FOOSH mechanism. This evaluation comprises a few specific tests.

The best-known test is for tenderness in the anatomic snuffbox (ASB). This is the depression formed by the borders of the radial styloid, the extensor pollicis longus tendon, and the paired extensor pollicis brevis and abductor pollicis longus tendons. The scaphoid is located on the "floor" of this triangular depression (see Figure 3.2). Another important test is axial compression (AC) of the scaphoid. The thumb is held gently in mid-abduction and extension, and force is directed toward the base of the thumb. A less commonly applied, but more accurate, test [21] is palpation for tenderness of the scaphoid tubercle (ST). This prominence of the distal scaphoid is found on the volar aspect of the wrist, along the distal wrist flexor crease, about one centimeter ulnarly from the radial styloid. The tubercle becomes more prominent in radial deviation, and disappears in ulnar deviation.

Combining the tests will increase the accuracy. Two studies have found that while both the ASB and AC tests are 100% sensitive, the AC is much more specific [22, 21]. Furthermore, one study found that

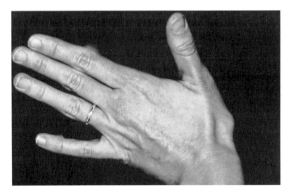

Figure 3.2 The anatomic snuffbox (ASB). The ASB is the depression formed by the borders of the radial styloid, the extensor pollicis longus tendon, and the paired extensor pollicis brevis and abductor pollicis longus tendons.

diagnosis based on tenderness with all three tests greatly increased specificity without sacrificing sensitivity [21]. Nonetheless, many acute care providers elect to consider a positive finding on any of these tests as evidence for a presumptive fracture.

Given a history and physical examination that suggests an injury, the acute care provider should obtain imaging of the scaphoid. In the vast majority of cases the initial evaluation will utilize plain radiographs.

If the initial radiographs are negative, the first consideration is to determine if the appropriate films were obtained. A standard series of wrist radiographs will comprise AP and lateral views. It is important to consider that the scaphoid will appear in an oblique position on these views, however, making it more difficult to identify a fracture. The scaphoid view, an AP view with the wrist held in ulnar deviation, will rotate the scaphoid into a plane perpendicular to the x-ray beam, and will reveal subtle fractures. Despite an optimal set of negative radiographs, a small percentage of those patients with a concerning history and examination will be shown to have a fracture at follow-up. This number is generally thought to be about 15%.

If a fracture is found on the initial films, the degree of displacement should be determined. If there is any degree of displacement, consultation with a hand surgeon is needed, as this will require surgical management. If there is no displacement, the patient may be discharged with a long-arm thumb spica splint. An outpatient evaluation by a hand surgeon should be arranged, as surgical management, especially for proximal fractures, may be preferable to prolonged casting.

If no fracture is found, but the examination is concerned about an occult fracture, the common practice is to place the patient in a short-arm thumb spica cast, and arrange for re-evaluation and repeat radiographs in 10 days. These may show sclerosis of the fracture line, or other subtle, indirect signs of healing.

> KEY FACT | **Approximately 15% of patients with a history and examination concerning for scaphoid fracture and negative radiographs will have a fracture at follow-up.**

Pitfall | **Failure to consider clenched-fist injury during evaluation of a wound to the hand**

Even when dealing with the prosaic cutaneous wound, the acute care provider must be meticulous in their evaluation and treatment. These consider-ations are all the more important when dealing with wounds to the hand caused by striking another person in the teeth, known as a clenched-fist injury (CFI), or more colloquially, a "fight bite."

The stereotypical patient who presents to the ED with a fight bite is a young male. Often, the patient will present more than a day after the injury, and may be showing frank signs of infection [23]. Although the injury is often associated with alcohol consumption, there is a tendency on the part of the patient to avoid being candid about the nature of the injury. One prospective study found that many patients coming to the ED with a wound do not ini-tially volunteer the cause as a human bite.

Consecutive patients presenting to a Scottish ED had a formatted history recorded by the treating physician. Patients who did not volunteer a history of a bite injury were asked a scripted prompt during the initial evaluation. A total of 100 patients were identified as having suffered a human bite, either a

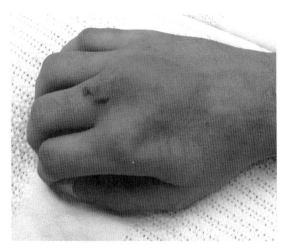

Figure 3.3 Fight bite. This patient presented 12 hours after a fight bite. Note the innocuous appearing wound over the MCP joint. (Courtesy Dr Lauren Tobias.)

CFI or an occlusion injury, during the study period. 62 patients volunteered such a history, but the use of the direct prompt in the interview was necessary in 38 of the 100 patients. This subset of patients tended to be those who had suffered a CFI (as opposed to an occlusion injury), presented late, or who had presented with an infected wound [24].

> KEY FACT | **The addition of a direct prompt in the interview to elicit the history of a bite wound was necessary in 38% of the subjects.**

It behooves the acute care provider to suspect any wound of the hand to have been caused by a CFI mechanism.

A CFI is incurred when a flexed hand is struck against teeth, and will typically involve a wound overlying either the second or third metacar-pophalangeal (MCP) joints [23]. The wound may appear minor, with a laceration of under five milli-meters common [25]. The skin overlying the MCP is thin, and affords little protection of the relatively superficial tendons and MCP joint space. (See Figure 3.3)

The evaluation should be both clinical and radiologic. After a full neurovascular and musculo-skeletal exam of the hand and wrist, attention must be paid to creating optimal conditions for wound evaluation. Bright lights should be employed and the patient should have their hand positioned for easy examination. If bleeding obscures the view, a bloodless field should be assured. Because of the size of the typical laceration, one may need to extend the laceration to fully explore injured structures. A crucial consideration is that the wound must be examined in the position in which it was injured, i.e. fully flexed. A partially cut extensor tendon may be missed if the finger is examined in extension, as the injured portion of the tendon will be located proximal to the cutaneous wound. Similarly, the MCP joint should be examined with the joint in full flexion in order to investigate for the possibility of intra-articular injury.

> KEY FACT | **A crucial consideration is that the wound must be examined in the position in which it was injured, i.e. fully flexed. A partially injured extensor tendon may be missed if the finger is examined in extension.**

Radiographs of the joint should be obtained to look for retained tooth fragments or fractures of the metacarpal head or proximal phalanx. In the patient who presents with apparent infection, signs of osteomyelitis should also be sought. One ED-based study found that, out of 30 patients with a fight bite, 6 showed fractures of the MCP, the distal phalanx, or of the MCP head [23].

After careful examination, the wound should be copiously flushed with normal saline under pressure.

The wound should be left to heal by secondary intention. The hand should be splinted in the position of comfort and tetanus immunization should be addressed.

If there is no sign of injury beyond the skin, "prophylactic" antibiotics should be prescribed, and a recheck arranged for 24 hours later. Even in seemingly-innocuous wounds, antibiotics must be prescribed in human bite wounds, as the risk of subsequent infection is drastically decreased [26, 27]. Oral antibiotics should be active against the most common pathogens (e.g. streptococci, staphylococci, eikenella). Amoxicillin-clavulanate or a fluoroquinolone plus clindamycin are two acceptable regimens [28].

If there are signs of injury to the tendon or joint space, intravenous antibiotics should be given, and consultation made to a hand surgeon. Such patients may warrant admission, especially if there are signs of infection, or if there are any concerns about the patient's ability to follow-up. Patients with an infected CFI may be taken emergently to the operating room for further examination, debridement, and irrigation.

> KEY FACT | **Even in seemingly innocuous wounds, antibiotics must be prescribed in human bite wounds, as the risk of subsequent infection is drastically decreased.**

Pitfall | **Diagnosing an occult tendon injury as a "sprained" finger**

Many patients present to an urgent care center after having suffered an injury to a finger. While the eventual diagnosis in many of these patients will be that of a simple "sprain" or "jammed finger," with a benign prognosis, the inadequate evaluation, diagnosis, and management of certain conditions could predispose the patient to long-term disability.

Central slip tear

The extensors of the finger comprise of the central slip tendon, which inserts onto the proximal middle phalanx, and the paired lateral band tendons, which insert onto the proximal distal phalanx.

A mechanism that involves the forcible flexion of an actively extended PIPJ may cause the central slip tendon to partially or fully tear. Less frequently, such a tear can result from a volar dislocation of the PIPJ. Both these mechanisms could also produce a "mallet" finger, and the suspicion of one injury should prompt an examination for the other [29].

Initially, such an injury may be difficult to diagnose. In addition to the obstacles that pain and swelling present to examination, weakness of extension of the PIPJ may be occult because the action of the lateral bands can compensate. Even with a complete central slip tendon tear, the patient may be able to extend the PIPJ [30]. Eventually,

(a)

(b)

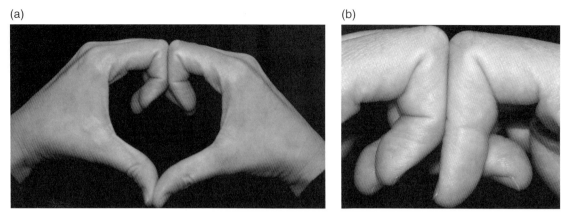

Figure 3.4 Modified Elson test. (a) The modified Elson test is performed by asking the patient to place the dorsal aspects of the middle phalanges of the injured finger and the same finger of the opposite side together with the proximal interphalangeal joints flexed to 90 degrees. The patient is asked to push the fingers together while trying to extend the DIP joint of both fingers. (b) The finger with the central slip injury will extend more at the DIP joint.

however, those lateral bands will subluxate in a palmar direction, producing the characteristic "boutonnière" deformity. Delay in diagnosis may preclude surgical repair and appropriate physical therapy to allow for a good functional outcome.

> KEY FACT | **Even with a complete central slip tendon tear, the patient may be able to extend the proximal interphalangeal joint (PIPJ).**

Examination may reveal maximal tenderness at the dorsal PIPJ, as well as a loss of active ROM and strength in extension [7, 31]. The accuracy of the examination may be enhanced with certain techniques. A test described by Elson [32], or a variant of that test [33], may be used to "isolate" the central slip. (See Figure 3.4.)

If the PIPJ joint is held flexed at 90°, the tension of the loaded central slip prevents extensor action along the lateral bands. If the central slip is torn, however, the lateral bands can be tensioned, and the distal interphalangeal joint (DIPJ) extended. A recent modification of the test involves apposing the dorsal surface of the middle phalanx of the injured finger against the dorsal surface of the contralateral middle phalanx. The degree of extension is easily compared between the injured and uninjured fingers [33].

If a central slip injury is suspected, the PIPJ should be splinted in extension for four weeks, but with the DIPJ and MCP joints left mobile. This position is essential to preventing palmar subluxation of the lateral extensor bands, and subsequent development of a boutonnière deformity [34]. Patients should be urgently referred to a hand surgeon if there is fracture of any size associated with the tendon injury, as they require open reduction and internal fixation [35].

> KEY FACT | **Splint the PIPJ in full extension, with the MCP and distal joints left mobile.**

Jersey finger

An avulsion of the flexor digitorum profundus (FDP) tendon can result in significant disability if diagnosis and management is delayed. Acute injuries are typically of the ring finger, and involve forced extension of a flexed DIPJ. The colloquial names for this injury, "jersey" and "rugger's" finger refer a common precipitating event; a rugby or football player, grabbing with a flexed finger at another player's jersey, only to have their finger forcibly pulled away.

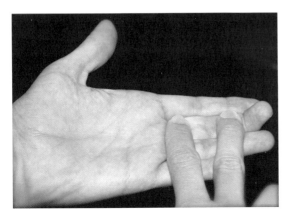

Figure 3.5 FDP test. To isolate the flexion of the FDP, the patient is ask to flex the finger at the DIP joint while the PIP joint and MCP joint are held in extension.

This flexor tendon has its weakest point just distal to the insertion on the volar base of the distal phalanx [36]. About half of these injuries will also have a small concomitant bony avulsion. Such a bony fragment may limit proximal retraction of the tendon, and thus also limit damage to the vincula that attach to the tendon, and serve to deliver blood flow. Without a bony fragment, the torn tendon may retract distally much further, and the subsequent risk of developing contractures is much higher.

There will typically be significant tenderness or swelling at the DIP, but this is variable [31]. The path of the FDP should be palpated to determine the point of maximum tenderness, as this could represent the distal edge of the torn tendon. AP and lateral radiographs should be obtained, although injuries without a fracture, and thus at high risk of poor outcomes, will be invisible radiographically [34].

Flexion of the DIPJ needs to be assessed in a manner that isolates the action of the FDP. The injured finger is flexed at the DIPJ while the MCP and PIP joints are held in extension by the examiner. If the patient has diminished strength on this exam, a tendon avulsion should be assumed, and splinting and urgent referral arranged. (See Figure 3.5.)

| KEY FACT | **Flexion of the DIPJ needs to be assessed in a manner that isolates the action of the FDP.**

A splint should be applied before discharge. Apply a dorsal splint to the wrist and hand that maintains the wrist in 30 degrees of flexion, the MCP in 70 degrees of flexion, and the PIP and DIP joints in 30 degrees of flexion [31, 7].

Almost all injuries of the FDP will require operative management, with the best results obtained with acute presentations. Injuries without an associated avulsion fracture should have more urgent orthopedics follow-up, as surgical repair is typically preferred within 7 days.

Mallet finger

The injury that is commonly referred to as the "mallet finger" is a partial or total tear of the distal extensor tendon of the finger. This tear may involve only the tendon just proximal to the insertion on the base of the distal phalanx, or it may involve an associated bony avulsion.

The injury is classically described as a sports injury, but it is commonly caused secondary to household chores, and the trauma does not need to be severe [37, 26]. The mechanism requires an actively extended finger that receives a blow that forces the distal interphalangeal joint (DIPJ) into flexion.

While the middle finger is said to be theoretically most vulnerable to this injury, different series find varying rates of injury for each digit. The thumb and index fingers are rarely involved, while the third, fourth, and fifth fingers of the dominant hand are usually injured [37, 36].

The injury classically presents with a tender, swollen DIPJ, as well as an extensor lag; i.e. a slight flexion of the DIP while full active extension is attempted by the patient. The degree of tenderness is variable, and may be absent [31]. In addition, extensor lag may be masked through the action of the unaffected extensor central slip tendon, or may become evident only later. It is necessary to specifically examine the integrity of the DIPJ extensor tendon in isolation.

The ability to fully extend the DIPJ passively should also be assessed [34]. Radiographs, both AP and lateral, should be obtained.

Table 3.1 Evaluation and treatment of closed tendon injuries of the finger

Injury	Examination	Treatment
Central slip extensor tendon injury (boutonnière deformity)	Tender at dorsal aspect of the PIP joint (middle phalanx) Inability to actively extend the PIP joint. Abnormal Elson test	Splint the PIP joint in full extension for six weeks.
Extensor tendon injury at the DIP joint (mallet finger)	Tender at dorsal aspect of the DIP joint No active extension of the DIP joint Tender at volar aspect of the DIP joint	Splint the DIP joint continuously for six weeks.
FDP tendon injury (jersey finger)	Inability to flex the isolated DIP joint	Splint finger and refer to orthopedic or hand surgeon.

Adapted from Wasserman *et al.* [17] with permission from Elsevier.

> KEY FACT | **It is necessary to specifically examine the integrity of the DIPJ extensor tendon in isolation.**

Closed injuries to the distal extensor tendon, with or without a small (<25% of the articular surface) avulsion fracture should be splinted in full extension. The specific type of splint is not important [37], but compliance is paramount to achieving the best outcome. The DIPJ joint needs to be splinted in extension for six to eight weeks, without interruption. Any brief failure to maintain extension requires another six to eight weeks. Despite this, the risk of skin breakdown requires that the splint be removed daily for cleaning and drying. Failure to comply with the splinting regimen may result in a "swan-neck" deformity, due to unopposed action of the central slip tendon, and patients should be informed of this possibility [31].

Distal extensor tendon injuries that require referral to a hand surgeon include: avulsion >25% of articular surface, nontrivial soft tissue damage (lacerations, deep abrasion) [36, 34], inability to passively extend the DIPJ, and volar subluxation of the distal phalanx [34]. (See Table 3.1 for summary.)

Pearls for improving patient outcomes

• Obtain axillary view radiographs if a posterior shoulder dislocation is suspected.

• Patients with a possible septic bursitis should be reevaluated within 48–72 hours.

• If a scaphoid fracture is suspected, radiographs should include AP views of the wrist in ulnar deviation.

• Examine the CFI wound through the full ROM, most crucially with the MCP in full flexion.

• A mallet finger should be referred to a hand surgeon if an avulsion fracture exceeds 25% of the articular surface, there is significant soft tissue damage, the DIP joint cannot be passively extended, or there is a volar subluxation of the distal phalanx.

• Advise the patient with the mallet finger to remove the DIP joint extension splint daily in order to let the finger dry off. The finger should be kept flat on a table while the splint is off, and the patient should use assistance to re-splint.

• Perform a test to check for integrity of the central slip if a tear is suspected. Appose the dorsal surface of the middle phalanx of the injured finger against the dorsal surface of the contralateral middle phalanx. The test is positive if the DIPJ can be actively extended.

• A central slip tendon tear that is associated with a significant fracture should be urgently referred to a hand surgeon for early ORIF.

References

1 Huisstede BM, Bierma-Zeinstra SM, Koes BW, Verhaar JA. Incidence and prevalence of upper-extremity musculoskeletal disorders. A systematic appraisal of the literature. *BMC Musculoskelet Disord* 2006; **7**: 7.

2 Cicak N. Posterior dislocation of the shoulder. *J Bone Joint Surg, Br Vol* 2004; **86**(3): 324–332.

3 Kowalsky MS, Levine WN. Traumatic posterior glenohumeral dislocation: classification, pathoanatomy, diagnosis, and treatment. *Orthop Clin North Am* 2008; **39**(4): 519–533, viii.

4 Robinson CM, Aderinto J. Posterior shoulder dislocations and fracture-dislocations. *J Bone Joint Surg, Am Vol* 2005; **87**(3): 639–650.

5 Perron AD, Jones RL. Posterior shoulder dislocation: avoiding a missed diagnosis. *Am J Emerg Med* 2000; **18**(2): 189–191.

6 Mouzopoulos G. The "Mouzopoulos" sign: a radiographic sign of posterior shoulder dislocation. *Emerg Radiol* 2010; **17**(4): 317–320.

7 Simon RR, Koenigsknecht SJ. Chapter 11. Shoulder and arm; emergency orthopedics: The Extremities. *Emergency Orthopedics: The Extremities*: McGraw-Hill; 2007.

8 Small LN, Ross JJ. Suppurative tenosynovitis and septic bursitis. *Infect Dis Clin North Am* 2005; **19**(4): 991–1005, xi.

9 Zimmermann B, 3rd, Mikolich DJ, Ho G, Jr. Septic bursitis. *Semin Arthrit Rheumat* 1995; **24**(6): 391–410.

10 Martinez-Taboada VM, Cabeza R, Cacho PM, *et al.* Cloxacillin-based therapy in severe septic bursitis: retrospective study of 82 cases. *Joint Bone, Spine: Revue du Rhumat* 2009; **76**(6): 665–669.

11 Gaughan EM, Ritter ML, Kumar PN, Timpone JG. Serious infection from Staphylococcus aureus in 2 HIV-infected patients receiving fusion inhibitor therapy. *AIDS Reader* 2008; **18**(5): 266–268.

12 Murray RJ, Pearson JC, Coombs GW, *et al.* Outbreak of invasive methicillin-resistant Staphylococcus aureus infection associated with acupuncture and joint injection. *Infection Control and Hospital Epidemiology: The Official Journal of The Society of Hospital Epidemiologists of America* 2008; **29**(9): 859–865.

13 Stell IM. Management of acute bursitis: outcome study of a structured approach. *J Royal Soc Med* 1999; **92**(10): 516–521.

14 Stell IM, Gransden WR. Simple tests for septic bursitis: comparative study. *BMJ (Clinical research edn.)* 1998; **316**(7148): 1877.

15 Smith DL, McAfee JH, Lucas LM, *et al.* Treatment of nonseptic olecranon bursitis. A controlled, blinded prospective trial. *Arch Internal Med* 1989; **149**(11): 2527–2530.

16 Ho G, Jr., Tice AD. *Comparison of nonseptic and septic bursitis. Further observations on the treatment of septic bursitis. Arch Internal Med* 1979; **139**(11): 1269–1273.

17 Wasserman AR, Melville LD, Birkhahn RH. Septic bursitis: a case report and primer for the emergency clinician. *J Emerg Med* 2009 Oct; **37**(3): 269–272.

18 Cardone DA, Tallia AF. Diagnostic and therapeutic injection of the elbow region. *Am Fam Phys* 2002; **66**(11): 2097–2100.

19 Gilbert DN (ed.). *The Sanford Guide to Antimicrobial Therapy.* Antimicrobial Therapy, Inc.; 2010.

20 Perron AD, Brady WJ. Evaluation and management of the high-risk orthopedic emergency. *Emerg Med Clin North Am* 2003; **21**(1): 159–204.

21 Parvizi J, Wayman J, Kelly P, Moran CG. Combining the clinical signs improves diagnosis of scaphoid fractures. A prospective study with follow-up. *J Hand Surg (Edinburgh, Scotland).* 1998; **23**(3): 324–327.

22 Grover R. Clinical assessment of scaphoid injuries and the detection of fractures. *J Hand Surg (Edinburgh, Scotland)* 1996; **21**(3): 341–343.

23 Goon P, Mahmoud M, Rajaratnam, V. Hand trauma pitfalls: a retrospective study of fight bites. *Euro J Trauma Emerg Surg* 2008; **34**(2): 135–140.

24 Wallace CG, Robertson CE. Prospective audit of 106 consecutive human bite injuries: the importance of history taking. *Emerg Med J* 2005; **22**(12): 883–884.

25 Clark DC. Common acute hand infections. *Am Fam Phy.* 2003; **68**(11): 2167–2176.

26 Medeiros I, Saconato H. Antibiotic prophylaxis for mammalian bites. *Cochr Database Syst Rev* 2001(2): CD001738.

27 Zubowicz VN, Gravier M. Management of early human bites of the hand: a prospective randomized study. *Plastic Reconstruct Surg* 1991; **88**(1): 111–114.

28 Stevens DL, Bisno AL, Chambers HF, *et al.* Practice guidelines for the diagnosis and management of skin and soft-tissue infections. *Clin Infect Dis [An official publication of the Infectious Diseases Society of America]* 2005; **41**(10): 1373–1406.

29 Bindra RR, Foster BJ. Management of proximal interphalangeal joint dislocations in athletes. *Hand Clin* 2009; **25**(3): 423–435.

30 Rubin J, Bozentka DJ, Bora FW. Diagnosis of closed central slip injuries. A cadaveric analysis of non-invasive tests. *J Hand Surg (Edinburgh, Scotland)* 1996; **21**(5): 614–616.

31 Perron AD, Brady WJ, Keats TE, Hersh RE. Orthopedic pitfalls in the emergency department: closed tendon injuries of the hand. *Am J Emerg Med* 2001; **19**(1): 76–80.

32 Elson RA. Rupture of the central slip of the extensor hood of the finger. A test for early diagnosis. *J Bone Joint Surg, Br Vol* 1986; **68**(2): 229–231.

33 Venus M, Little C. The modified Elson's test in open central slip injury. *Injury Extra* 2010; **41**(11): 128–129.

34 Leggit JC, Meko CJ. Acute finger injuries: part I. Tendons and ligaments. *Am Fam Phys* 2006; **73**(5): 810–816.

35 Freiberg A, Pollard BA, Macdonald MR, Duncan MJ. Management of proximal interphalangeal joint injuries. *Hand Clin* 2006 Aug; **22**(3): 235–242.

36 Tuttle HG, Olvey SP, Stern PJ. Tendon avulsion injuries of the distal phalanx *Clin Ortho Related Res* 2006; **445**: 157–168.

37 Handoll HH, Vaghela MV. Interventions for treating mallet finger injuries. *Cochr Database System Rev (Online)* 2004; **3**(3): CD004574.

38 Roberts JR, Hedges JR, Chanmugam AS. Chapter 53 in: *Clinical Procedures in Emergency Medicine* (4th edn.). Philadelphia, PA: W.B. Saunders; 2004.

CHAPTER 4

Orthopedic Pitfalls of the Lower Extremity

Christopher S. Kiefer
Department of Emergency Medicine, Indiana University School of Medicine, Indianapolis, IN, USA

Introduction

Lower extremity injuries and pain are commonly encountered in clinical practice and account for 4.8% of all injury-related visits to Emergency Departments in the United States [1]. The majority of the presenting complaints can be safely and adequately managed in an urgent care setting, but the clinician must be vigilant in the evaluation of these patients in order to identify those in need of more extensive diagnostic testing, immediate referral to specialist care, or aggressive initial therapy.

Pitfall | Assuming that a swollen joint is caused by gout

Acute swelling and pain of a single joint in the lower extremity is a common presenting complaint to Urgent Care Centers. The differential diagnosis includes both gout and septic arthritis. Gout is a clinical entity characterized by the formation of monosodium urate crystals in the joint space leading to an acutely erythematous, warm, and painful joint. It most commonly involves the great toe, although any joint may be affected. Gout is a recognized cause of an acute monoarticular arthritis, but patients with an acutely swollen joint must be evaluated for potential septic arthritis, which, if ignored, could quickly lead to joint destruction.

Septic arthritis in a native joint generally occurs after hematogenous seeding of the joint during an episode of bacteremia. The bacteria enter the joint space, leading to an inflammatory reaction and associated subchondral bone destruction within a few days. Irreversible loss of function can occur in 25–50% of affected patients despite the initiation of antibiotics [2]. In addition, septic arthritis can lead to systemic manifestations including sepsis and death with an in-hospital mortality as high as 7–15% of affected patients [3]. Risk factors for developing septic arthritis are outlined in Box 4.1. The most commonly isolated organism is *Staphylococcus aureus*, including methicillin-resistant *S. aureus* (MRSA) [2].

When evaluating a patient with an acute monoarthritis, the clinician should begin with a careful history focusing on the duration of the arthritis, concurrent medical illnesses (acute and chronic), preceding trauma, fever, history of intravenous drug use, previous episodes, alcohol history, sexual activity, and immunosuppression. The presence in the history of fever, intravenous drug usage, multiple sexual partners and immunosuppression should increase suspicion of a possible infectious etiology. Physical examination should focus on the joint involved as well as an examination of the contralateral joint for comparison. Unfortunately, a recent meta-analysis revealed that history and physical examination alone do not reliably identify the underlying cause of an acute monoarthritis [4].

Urgent Care Emergencies: Avoiding the Pitfalls and Improving the Outcomes, First Edition.
Edited by Deepi G. Goyal and Amal Mattu.
© 2012 John Wiley & Sons, Ltd. Published 2012 by John Wiley & Sons, Ltd.

> **Box 4.1** Risk factors associated with an increased likelihood of septic arthritis
>
> Prosthetic joint
> Age >80 years
> Rheumatoid arthritis
> Overlying cellulitis
> History of trauma to the area over the joint
> Intravenous drug usage
> Immunosuppression
>
> Data from Margaretten *et al.* [3].

In an attempt to differentiate septic arthritis from other less devastating potential etiologies of an acutely swollen joint, clinicians will often obtain laboratory data, including a complete blood count, an erythrocyte sedimentation rate (ESR), and a C-reactive protein (CRP). Unfortunately, a normal test result does not rule out disease while an abnormal test result does not help in "ruling in" septic arthritis as was found in a study of 47 patients with confirmed septic arthritis. This study revealed that all patients had an elevated ESR and all but one patient had an elevated CRP. However, the systemic white blood cell WBC) count (was normal in 28/47 patients; including 50% of patients with concurrent rheumatoid arthritis and an acute septic arthritis [5]. While this study highlights problems with the sensitivity of these laboratory values, low specificity is another major limitation. One retrospective cohort study of patients with culture-proven septic arthritis found the specificity of the WBC count to be 55%, and the specificity of the ESR to be only 11%. Because of the poor diagnostic characteristics of these tests, they are of little value in evaluating the patient with an acutely swollen joint [3, 6].

Because gout is caused by urate crystals, it is logical to assume that a serum uric acid may help to identify those with gout. However, uric acid levels can be affected by multiple factors including diet and impaired urinary excretion. While having an elevated serum uric acid level can be a predictor of gouty arthritis [7], up to 33% of patients with an acute gout will have a normal serum uric acid level [8]. Therefore, the presence or absence of an ele-

vated serum uric acid level alone cannot adequately differentiate between gout and septic arthritis.

> KEY FACT | **An elevated serum uric acid level does not definitively establish the diagnosis of gout.**

The only way to reliably differentiate inflammatory from septic arthritis is to perform arthrocentesis and joint fluid analysis. While obtaining synovial fluid via arthrocentesis is the gold standard for differentiating these two entities, this may be beyond the capabilities of some urgent care centers. If synovial fluid is obtained, it should be sent for cell count and differential, Gram stain, culture, and crystal analysis. Regarding the synovial fluid WBC count, no definitive cutoff measurement to confirm the diagnosis of septic arthritis has been clearly established [6], although the likelihood of septic arthritis increases as the synovial WBC count increases. A synovial WBC count between 25,000 and 50,000 is associated with nearly a three times greater likelihood of septic arthritis, and a synovial WBC count greater than 50,000 is associated with a seven times greater likelihood of septic arthritis. An elevated synovial WBC count is likely to be the best predictor of potential septic arthritis while awaiting the culture [3].

Arthrocentesis will also provide analysis of any crystalline material present in the joint. The two major types of synovial crystals found are negatively birefringent uric acid crystals and positively birefringent calcium pyrophosphate crystals. The latter is suggestive of psuedogout; a condition that is managed very similarly to gout. If uric acid crystals are present in a synovial fluid sample, it is suggestive of gouty arthritis, but unfortunately cannot completely rule out the possibility of septic arthritis. A recent retrospective study demonstrated that 1.5% of all synovial fluid samples with crystals present ultimately have positive culture results, suggesting concomitant septic and gouty arthritis [9]. Although this is rare, it is important to remember that the presence of crystals does not completely exclude septic arthritis.

Ultimately, the presence or absence of septic arthritis will be determined by the synovial fluid culture, which will not be available at the time of initial evaluation. Given the potential for morbidity from treatment delays, those patients with predictors of septic arthritis present – a history of immunosuppression, history of prosthetic joint, elevated ESR/CRP, elevated synovial WBC count greater than 50,000, absence of crystalline disease on arthrocentesis – should be referred to an inpatient setting and have parenteral antibiotics administered while awaiting cultures.

> KEY FACT | Joint fluid analysis is required to definitively differentiate gout from septic arthritis.

Pitfall | Failure to consider gonococcal arthritis as the cause of an erythematous, swollen joint in a young, sexually active patient

Young sexually active patients without active urogenital complaints may present to an Urgent Care Center with low-grade fever, a rash, and joint pain. In this clinical scenario, the practitioner must be suspicious of disseminated gonococcal infection leading to gonococcal arthritis or tenosynovitis. *Neisseria gonorrhoeae* is a Gram-negative intracellular diplococcus that is transmitted through sexual contact. Initially, infection is established in the lower genital tract of both male and female patients, although some patients may be asymptomatic. Some strains of *Neisseria gonorrhoeae* are capable of dissemination, causing disease distant from the genital tract. Dissemination is more common in women than in men and classically occurs during menstruation and pregnancy. The rash is most commonly described as an erythematous maculopapular eruption, although other skin lesions including vesicles, bullae, erythema multiforme, and urticaria may be seen. In contrast to nongonococcal septic arthritis, gonococcal arthritis is more likely to involve smaller joints including the ankle, wrist, fingers, and toes. It also tends to be asymmetric. It is important to keep in mind that the patient may not present with an overtly swollen joint suggestive of a suppurative arthritis and present instead with a tenosynovitis. The practitioner must maintain a high index of suspicion, as the diagnosis can again be fraught with difficulty based upon the initial presentation and laboratory studies.

In those patients presenting with gonococcal arthritis, synovial culture will demonstrate *N. gonorrhea* in only 25–50% [10, 11], making it necessary to also obtain cultures from sites traditionally affected by *N. gonorrhoeae* – the cervix in females, the urethra in males, the rectum, and the posterior pharynx. In addition, synovial WBC count will often be less than 50,000 [11]. Despite the fact that patients with disseminated gonococcal infection may not report symptoms in the anogenital tract or posterior pharynx, gonococcal infection will be identified in one of these areas in 70–80% of patients [12]. As with septic arthritis, patients with gonococcal arthritis should be admitted to an inpatient setting for administration of parenteral antibiotics.

> KEY FACT | Synovial cultures will be positive for *Neisseria gonorrhoeae* in only 25–50% of patients with gonococcal arthritis.

Pitfall | Failure to diagnose a fibular head fracture in a patient presenting with ankle pain

Most acute care providers will encounter a patient with an ankle injury on nearly every shift. The provider should begin evaluation of these patients with a careful history and physical examination, with a focus on the mechanism of injury; the time elapsed since the injury, the direction of stress placed on the ankle (inversion, eversion, forced dorsiflexion, forced plantar flexion), and the ability of the patient to bear weight. After assessing any obvious deformity of the ankle, the provider should check for the dorsalis pedis and posterior tibial pulses, the patient's ability to plantar and dorsiflex the foot, and tenderness to palpation at the following landmarks: medial malleolus, lateral malleolus, head of the fifth metatarsal, and fibular head. The Ottawa Ankle Rules (Figure 4.1) have been validated as a clinical decision-making guide with regards as to when to obtain plain radiographs of the ankle. These rules were developed to

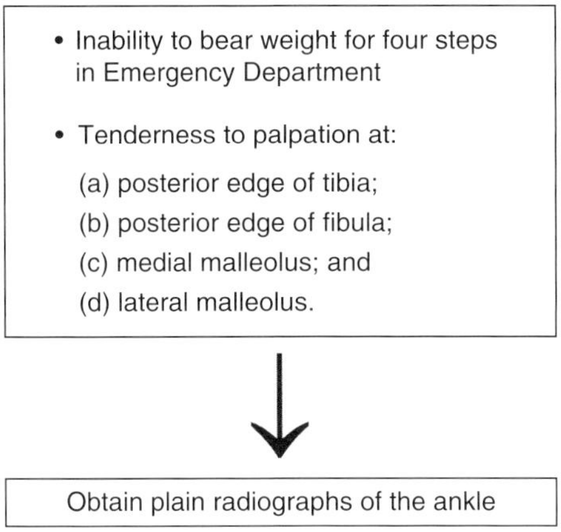

- Inability to bear weight for four steps in Emergency Department

- Tenderness to palpation at:

  (a) posterior edge of tibia;

  (b) posterior edge of fibula;

  (c) medial malleolus; and

  (d) lateral malleolus.

Obtain plain radiographs of the ankle

Figure 4.1 The Ottawa Ankle Rules are a clinical decision rule to guide clinicians in determining which patients require plain radiographs of the ankle to be obtained. (Data from Stiell *et al.* [26].)

minimize unnecessary radiography and have a sensitivity approaching 100% for ankle fracture [13]. They can be safely used to differentiate those patients at risk for fracture versus those patients with an isolated ankle sprain who may be safely dismissed without imaging.

In those patients whom the Ottawa Ankle Rules would recommend ankle radiographs, the clinician should pay special attention to palpation of the fibular head. Maisonneuve's deformity is a fracture of the distal tibia at the ankle with extension of the injury through the interosseous membrane resulting in a fracture of the proximal third of the fibula. Patients may complain only of ankle pain, making it essential to palpate the head of the fibula. If the fibular head is tender, radiographs of the tibia and fibula should also be obtained, as standard trauma views of the ankle will fail to detect the fracture in the proximal fibula. Failure to diagnose this fracture can result in long-term sequelae, including arthritis and limitation of daily activities secondary to pain [14].

If a Maisonneuve's deformity is detected, urgent care management will consist of placing the patient in a well-formed, well-padded posterior slab splint from the level of the popliteal fossa to the toes. The patient should be referred to an Orthopedic Surgeon as an outpatient for definitive casting and potential surgical management.

Pitfall | **Failure to consider Achilles tendon rupture in an ambulatory patient.**

While evaluating a patient with an acutely injured ankle or lower extremity, it is essential to evaluate the Achilles tendon for potential injury. The Achilles tendon is located in the posterior aspect of the calf and serves to connect the gastrocnemius and soleus muscles to the calcaneus. Achilles tendon rupture predominately affects middle-aged men participating in athletic activities, and while its presence may be obvious to the acute care provider in certain cases, up to 25% of patients may present similarly to a simple sprained ankle and the rupture will be missed on an initial evaluation [15]. The key historical issues and examination findings the clinician should focus upon are the mechanism of injury, location of the pain, history of hearing a "popping sound," ability of the patient to plantar flex the foot, ability of the patient to ambulate, presence of a deformity over the posterior calf, and performance of the Thompson test to evaluate the Achilles tendon.

In patients presenting with an acute Achilles rupture, the majority will be asymptomatic prior to rupture. The patient will often report sudden pain associated with a "popping" sensation or sound after an attempt to rapidly accelerate or jump. The patient often will be unable to ambulate following the injury, but this is not absolute. During the evaluation in the Urgent Care Center, the patient's pain may have lessened or completely resolved. The patient may have preserved but limited ability to ambulate and to plantar flex the lower extremity due to the intact function of tibialis posterior, peroneal, and plantaris muscles [15].

KEY FACT | **Patients with an Achilles tendon rupture may still be able to ambulate and actively dorsiflex the affected lower extremity.**

In order to evaluate the Achilles tendon, the patient should be placed in the prone position with the ankles hanging off of the end of the gurney or examination table. In patients presenting with Achilles tendon rupture, there may be an obvious deformity when comparing one extremity to the other. However, hematoma formation following acute rupture may make the extremities appear roughly symmetric. In order to further evaluate the integrity of the tendon, the Thompson test should be performed with the patient in the prone position. The examiner should squeeze the calf gently and observe the affected extremity for the presence of plantar flexion in response to the squeeze. The presence of partial plantar flexion implies partial integrity of the tendon, while a lack of plantar flexion suggests tendon rupture. This test has been shown to have a sensitivity of 92% in patients with surgically proven Achilles tendon tears [16]. For patients with an equivocal Thompson test and high clinical suspicion for acute tendon rupture, other modalities such as a Copeland test can be employed. The patient should remain in the prone position, but flexed at the knee, while a blood pressure cuff is placed around the patient's calf and inflated to 100 mmHg. Then, the examiner should place the patient's ankle in plantar flexion. If the tendon is intact, the cuff will record an increase in pressure of 30–40 mmHg. If the tendon is injured, the measured pressure will not increase. Unfortunately, the utility of this diagnostic test is limited at times by patient discomfort and its reported sensitivity of approximately 80% [16].

In cases where the diagnosis remains uncertain following careful physical examination, radiographic studies including MRI, CT, and ultrasound may be performed, but they are generally not needed to establish the diagnosis. Patients diagnosed with an Achilles tendon tear should be splinted in plantar flexion and referred for prompt outpatient orthopedic evaluation.

Pitfall | Failure to identify a Lisfranc fracture-dislocation on plain radiographs of the foot

Acute care providers must consider the possibility of a Lisfranc fracture-dislocation of the tarsometatarsal joint in every patient presenting with a swollen, painful foot following trauma. The tarsometatarsal joint represents the junction of the forefoot and midfoot, with the osseous struc-

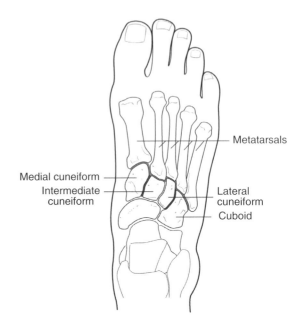

Figure 4.2 Bones of the Lisfranc (tarsometatarsal joint). (Courtesy of Sharon Teal. Reproduced with permission from Indiana University School of Medicine Office of Visual Media.)

tures consisting of the bases of the five metatarsals, the three cuneiform bones, and the cuboid. Transverse ligaments connect the bases of the second through fifth metatarsals while the Lisfanc ligament connects the medial cuneiform to the base of the second metatarsal [17]. Figure 4.2 illustrates the anatomic relationships of the bony structures forming the tarsometatarsal joint. The joint as a whole helps to maintain stability of the midfoot.

One commonly described mechanism of a Lisfranc injury is a direct blow to the foot with a significant axial load, which might occur in a motor vehicle accident or a fall from a height. The other common mechanism of injury is a longitudinal force applied to a plantar flexed foot. Physical examination findings may be variable, however; there is generally a marked amount of swelling and pain in the midfoot. Some patients will be completely unable to bear weight whereas others will have a relatively preserved ability to ambulate despite significant pain. The acute care provider should palpate for tenderness along the tarsometa-tarsal joint, which, if present, suggests underlying injury. The clinician should also assess for pain while passively pronating and abducting the fore-foot with the midfoot flexed. Performing this maneuver guides the patient's foot in a circle. The plantar surface of the foot should be examined carefully, as the presence of plantar ecchymosis should heighten the acute care provider's suspicion of a tarsometatarsal joint injury [18].

If there is suspicion of a Lisfranc injury following physical examination and history, plain radiography utilizing anterior–posterior, lateral, and oblique views should be obtained. The practitioner should use caution when considering whether to place an ACE type bandage prior to the patient having radio-graphs obtained. Placement of an ACE wrap may unintentionally reduce the fracture-dislocation and produce falsely negative images. However, up to 19% of patients with a Lisfranc injury will have neg-ative initial radiographs [19]. If these standard views are unable to clearly identify an injury, but one's clinical suspicion remains high, weight-bearing views should be obtained as some Lisfranc fractures are only visible on a weight-bearing view [20].

> KEY FACT | **Up to 19% of patients with a Lisfranc injury will have negative initial radiographs.**

Still, the majority of Lisfranc fracture-dislocations will be readily apparent on initial studies. When evaluating radiographs for evidence of a subtle Lisfranc injury, the clinician should evaluate the metatarsals for the presence of fractures at the base of the second metatarsal, the cuneiforms, or the cuboid, as these are suggestive of injury to the tar-sometatarsal joint. In addition, providers should pay close attention to the relationship between the metatarsals and the cuneiform bones. On the AP and oblique views, the medial margins of the sec-ond metatarsal and the middle cuneiform should form a straight line. In addition, there should be a straight line between the medial border of the fourth metatarsal and the medial border of the cuboid bone [18].

Identifying a Lisfranc fracture-dislocation is essential in order to maximize patient recovery with intact function and without long-term compli-cations including arthritis. Once identified in the urgent care setting, the patient should be trans-ferred to a facility capable of obtaining a prompt orthopedic consultation in order to allow closed reduction of the injury and evaluation for immediate complications including compartment syndrome.

> KEY FACT | **Patients with Lisfranc fracture-dislocations are at risk for compartment syndrome.**

Pitfall | **Failing to differentiate between avulsion fractures of the fifth metatarsal and Jones fracture of the fifth metatarsal**

In patients presenting to the Urgent Care Center after trauma to their foot and ankle, it is essential to palpate over the fifth metatarsal on physical exam-ination, as this is the most commonly injured meta-tarsal bone in the acute care setting [21]. If the provider can elicit tenderness over the fifth meta-tarsal, radiographic views of the foot should be obtained. Acute care practitioners must be able to recognize avulsion fractures of the proximal fifth metatarsal, in which stress transmitted to the pero-neus brevis tendon separates a proximal bone fragment from the rest of the fifth metatarsal. Practitioners must differentiate this injury from a fracture at the junction of the diaphysis and metaphysis of the fifth metatarsal, commonly known as a Jones fracture. The mechanism of injury can be helpful in making this differentiation. Avulsion fractures tend to occur following ankle inversion with the foot in plantar flexion. A Jones fracture results from a vertical or mediolateral stress on the foot while in plantar flexion and the patient's weight centered over the lateral aspect of the fifth metatarsal [22].

In the event that plain radiography reveals an isolated avulsion fracture of the fifth metatarsal, the patient may be managed by allowing him/her to weight bear as tolerated in a hard-soled shoe with a referral for outpatient follow-up with an orthopedic surgeon. The majority of fifth meta-tarsal avulsion fractures will not require any additional treatment beyond this conservative approach.

Unfortunately, patients with a Jones fracture of the fifth metararsal do not share this benign prognosis. Jones fractures are prone to malunion or nonunion, as this area of the fifth metatarsal lies in a watershed area with regards to blood supply. In addition, the fifth metatarsal has the widest range of motion of the metatarsals, which can further complicate healing [21]. In order to minimize potential complications, these patients should be placed in a long-leg posterior splint and made non-weight bearing until follow-up with an orthopedic surgeon can be made on an outpatient basis.

> KEY FACT │ **Jones fracture of the fifth metatarsal is prone to nonunion and malunion and it is essential that these patients be properly immobilized and non-weight bearing.**

Pitfall │ **Failing to properly diagnose and provide appropriate referral for a patient with an acutely injured knee**

Many patients present to Urgent Care Centers following a traumatic knee injury. As with the other injury patterns described above, the evaluation of the patient should begin with a detailed history and physical examination. Special attention should be paid to the mechanism of injury and/or the presence of a "popping sound." The physical examination should focus upon the pattern of bony tenderness, the presence or absence of a joint effusion, and performance of the Lachman's test to evaluate ligamentous stability.

In the urgent care setting, magnetic resonance imaging (MRI) is unlikely to be available and is not indicated in the immediate management of acute knee injuries. Similar to ankle injuries, the Ottawa Knee Rules (Figure 4.3) have been validated in order to help clinicians in the efficient use of plain radiography. These rules identify situations where x-rays are more likely to be diagnostic and to help to limit unnecessary radiography. Plain radiography

---

If any of the following are present:

- Age > 55 years
- Isolated tenderness at the patella
- Tenderness at the fibular head
- Inability to flex the knee to 90 degrees
- Inability to bear weight for four steps immediately after injury or in the Emergency Department

Obtain plain radiographs of the knee

Figure 4.3 The Ottawa Knee Rule is a clinical decision rule intended to guide clinicians to those patients requiring plain radiographs of the knee. (Data from Stiell *et al.* [27].)

---

will not demonstrate any of the ligamentous structures, but can demonstrate significant soft tissue swelling, a joint effusion, or any fracture. Plain radiography will also help to evaluate the proximal tibia for the presence of a tibial plateau fracture.

Patients will often be concerned about meniscal or ligamentous injury. An anterior cruciate ligament (ACL) tear is suggested by a "popping" sound at the time of injury, presence of a joint effusion, and positive Lachman's test (increased laxity with anterior force applied to the knee and tibia). Unfortunately, acute care providers have difficulty recognizing acute ACL injuries from only historical and examination factors, with a recent Emergency Department study showing that only 7 out of 27 ACL tears were accurately diagnosed by emergency physicians [23]. Given the limitations of history and physical examination in the acute care setting, patients with a potential or suspected ACL injury should be placed in a knee immobilizer and referred to a sports medicine or orthopedic specialist. Clinicians prescribing knee immobilizers should be aware that atrophy of the quadriceps musculature can occur quickly. Patients should be instructed to remove the brace several times daily to exercise the quadriceps and hamstring muscles. In addition, clinicians should advise patients that the knee immobilizer is only for short-term use, and follow-up with the appropriate specialist is still needed.

> KEY FACT | **It is difficult for acute care providers to accurately diagnose the acutely injured knee; with the majority of ACL tears being missed by acute care providers based upon history and physical examination.**

The medial meniscus can be injured when an individual undergoes a sudden twisting of the knee. These patients will not present with a joint effusion and are not likely to hear a "popping sound." Classically, they present with acute knee pain and may report a sensation that the knee is "locking" [24]. The physical examination should include assessment for effusion, bony tenderness, and ligamentous laxity as described above. In addition, a McMurray test should be performed to specifically evaluate the medial meniscus. With the knee held in flexion, the examiner's hand is placed on the lateral aspect of the knee to provide stability. The examiner then externally rotates the knee while extending it. The presence of a click suggests a medial meniscal injury. Unfortunately, as is the case with ACL tears, injuries of the medial meniscus can be difficult to detect on physical examination alone. Only 53% of medial meniscus injuries will be diagnosed if the acute care practitioner relies upon a positive McMurray test [25]. Because of this poor sensitivity, a patient with a suspected or potential meniscal injury should also be placed in a knee immobilizer with the precautions described above, until they can have follow-up with a sports medicine or orthopedic specialist.

Pearls for improving patient outcomes
• Patients with a joint effusion should undergo arthrocentesis to rule out septic arthritis.
• In patients presenting to the urgent care setting with an ankle injury, acute care providers must palpate the proximal fibula in order to avoid missing Maisonneuve's deformity, which requires different treatment and disposition than an ankle sprain or isolated fracture.
• Acute care providers have difficulty in accurately differentiating between etiologies of an acutely injured knee. Patients presenting with an acutely injured knee should be placed in a knee immobilizer until evaluation by an orthopedic surgeon or sports medicine specialist.
• The Ottawa Knee and Ankle Rules, when applied appropriately, can assist acute care practitioners in identifying those patients in need of radiography, thereby reducing unnecessary studies.
• Loss of the anatomic relationships between the medial aspect of the second metatarsal and middle cuneiform, as well as loss of the relationship between the medial aspect of the fourth metatarsal and cuboid on plain radiographs, should raise the suspicion of a Lisfranc injury.

References

1 Nawar EW, Niska RW, Xu, J. National Hospital Ambulatory Medical Care Survey: 2005 Emergency Department Survey. *Adv Data Vital Hlth Statis* 2007 June 29; **386**: 1–32.
2 Goldenberg DL. Septic arthritis. *Lancet* 1998; **351**: 197–202.
3 Margaretten ME, Kowhles J, Moore D, Bent S. Does this adult patient have septic arthritis? *JAMA* 2007; **297**: 1478–1488.
4 Ma L, Cranney A, Holroyd-Leduc JM. Acute monoarthritis: What is the cause of my patient's swollen joint? *CMAJ* 2009; **180**: 59–64.
5 Gupta MN, Sturrock RD, Field M. A prospective 2 year study of 75 patients with adult-onset septic arthritis. *Rheumatology* 2001; **40**: 24–30.
6 Li SF, Cassidy C, Chang C, *et al*. Diagnostic utility of laboratory testing in septic arthritis. *Emerg Med J* 2007; **24**: 75–77.
7 Eggebeen AT. Gout: an update. *Am Family Phys* 2007; **76**: 801–808; 811–812.
8 Richette P, Bardin T. Gout. *Lancet* 2010; **375**: 318–328.
9 Shah K, Spear J, Nathanson L, *et al*. Does the presence of crystal arthritis rule out septic arthritis? *J Emerg Med* 2007; **32**: 23–26.
10 Shirtliff ME, Mader JT. Acute septic arthritis. *Clin Microbiol Rev* 2002; **15**: 527–544.

11 Zink BJ. Bone and joint infections. In: Marx JA, Hockberger RS, Walls RM, *et al.* (eds.), *Rosen's Emergency Medicine: Concepts and Clinical Practice* (6th edn.). Elsevier: Philadelphia, 2006: pp. 2190–2191.

12 Rice PA. Gonococcal arthritis. *Infec Dis Clin North Am* 2005; **19**: 853–861.

13 Bachmann L, Kolb E, Koller MT, *et al.* Accuracy of the Ottawa ankle rules to exclude fractures of the ankle and mid-foot: systematic review. *BMJ* 2003; **326**: 417.

14 Millen JC, Lindberg D. Maisonneuve fracture. *J Emerg Med*. Article in Press. Retrieved 11 January 2011.

15 Ufberg J, Harrigan RA, Cruz T, *et al.* Orthopedic pitfalls in the ED: Achilles rupture. *Am J Emerg Med* 2004; **22**: 596–600.

16 Maffulli N. The clinical diagnosis of subcutaneous tear of the Achilles tendon: a prospective study in 174 patients. *Am J Sports Med* 1998; **26**: 266–270.

17 Gupta RT, Wadwha RP, Learch TJ, *et al.* Lisfranc injury: imaging findings for this important but often-missed diagnosis. *Curr Probl Diagn Radiol* 2008; **37**: 115–126.

18 Perron AD, Brady WJ, Keats TE. Orthopedic pitfalls in the ED: Lisfranc fracture-dislocation. *Am J Emerg Med* 2001; **19**: 71–75.

19 Sherief TI, Muchi B, Greiss M. Lisfranc injury: how frequently does it get missed? And how can we improve? *Injury* 2007; **38**: 856–860.

20 Arntz CT, Veith RG, Hansen ST. Fractures and fracture-dislocations of the tarsometatarsal joint. *J Joint Bone Surg* 1988; **70**: 173–181.

21 Zwitser EW, Breederveld RS. Fractures of the fifth metatarsal; diagnosis and treatment. *Injury* 2010; **41**: 555–562.

22 Hatch RL, Alsobrook JA, Clugston JR. Diagnosis and management of metatarsal fractures. *Am Family Phys* 2007; **76**: 817–826.

23 Guillodo Y, Rannou N, Dubrana F, *et al.* Diagnosis of anterior cruciate ligament rupture in an Emergency Department. *J Trauma* 2008; **65**: 1078–1082.

24 Calmbach WL, Hutchens M. Evaluation of patients presenting with knee pain: part II differential diagnosis. *Am Fam Phys* 2003; **68**: 917–922.

25 Strayer RJ, Lang ES. Does this patient have a torn meniscus or ligament of the knee? *Ann Emerg Med* 2006; **47**: 499–501.

26 Stiell IG, Greenberg GH, McKnight RD, *et al.* Decision rules for the use of radiography in acute ankle injuries. *JAMA* 1993; **269**: 1127–1132.

27 Stiell IG, Wells GA, Hoag RH, *et al.* Implementation of the Ottawa knee rule for the use of radiography in acute knee injuries. *JAMA* 1997; **278**: 2075–2079.

CHAPTER 5
Orthopedic Pitfalls: Pediatrics

Jana L. Anderson and James L. Homme

Department of Emergency Medicine and Pediatrics, Mayo Clinic, Rochester, MN, USA

Introduction

Pediatric orthopedic injuries are challenging both in diagnosis and disposition. Young children are frequently difficult to examine due to their anxiety and underlying pain from the injury. In many instances, the exact mechanism for the injury is unknown yet one must always consider abuse. Pediatric joints differ from those of an adult in that a child's ligaments are stronger than the bone. This leaves the relatively weak cartilaginous growth plate as the area of least resistance resulting in a fracture rather than a sprain. Given the difficulty with the history, physical examination and radiologic evaluation of children, one must be diligent to avoid the pitfalls in pediatric orthopedics.

Pitfall | **Missing a growth plate fracture**

Pediatric fractures frequently involve shearing or torsional forces, resulting in fracture through the cartilaginous growth plate (physis). Nearly a third of pediatric fractures involve the growth plate [1]. Most commonly this occurs in the distal tibia or distal radius. The Salter–Harris (SH) classification system is used to describe growth plate fractures (Table 5.1) [2]. The likelihood of growth plate arrest increases with progression of the SH type; from 2 to 3% for SH type 1 fracture to 13% of SH type 4 fracture. SH type 5 fractures are the result of

severe impaction injury that typically is diagnosed in hindsight when growth arrest is detected. On a radiographically positive SH type 1 fracture, there will be a slight widening of the growth plate with no other visible bony abnormalities (Figure 5.1). This finding can be subtle. Therefore, any patient with tenderness at the growth plate following trauma should be treated for a possible fracture regardless of the x-ray findings. Management defers depending on the clinical suspicion of fracture. If suspicion is high, the child should be splinted and referred to orthopedics for casting and follow-up. If clinical suspicion is low, the child may remain in a splint for 2 weeks, and follow-up with their primary care physician. At follow-up, if the child has continued pain at the physis, or healing callus formation at the growth plate on repeat x-ray, the child should be referred to orthopedics for casting and follow-up.

> KEY FACT | **A child with point tenderness at his/her growth plate should be splinted and treated as if fractured, regardless of x-ray findings.**

Pitfall | **Missing a buckle fracture in a child with arm use and minimal pain after a fall**

A buckle, or torus, fracture of the distal forearm is the most common of all childhood extremity

---

Urgent Care Emergencies: Avoiding the Pitfalls and Improving the Outcomes, First Edition.
Edited by Deepi G. Goyal and Amal Mattu.
© 2012 John Wiley & Sons, Ltd. Published 2012 by John Wiley & Sons, Ltd.

Table 5.1 Salter–Harris classification of pediatric fractures

Type	Description	Mnemonic **SALTR**
1	Fracture through the growth plate	**S**ame (no change in x-ray)
2	Fracture through growth plate and away from the joint space (toward the metaphysis)	**A**way (from the joint)
3	Fracture through growth plate and towards the joint space (toward the epiphysis)	**L**ower (into the joint)
4	Fracture through both epiphysis and metaphysis, transecting the growth plate	**T**hrough both (above and lower)
5	Complete impaction of growth plate, usually not detected until growth arrest becomes apparent	**R**est (of the bone)

Data from Salter and Harris [2].

fractures. This type of fracture typically results from a fall onto an outstretch hand (FOOSH) mechanism. The force of impact causes a compression of the junction between the porous metaphysis and

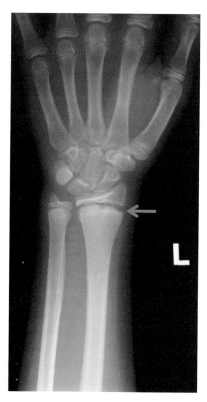

Figure 5.1 Salter–Harris type 1 fracture of the distal radius in a 9-year-old female. Note the slight widening of the growth plate of the radius (arrow).

the denser diaphysis of the child's forearm, causing buckling of the cortex. Though this type of fracture is at low risk for complications, accurate diagnosis is important for pain control by splinting and to prevent repeat visits for the same complaint. Children with this type of fracture may only have point tenderness at the fracture site. One must keep a high clinical suspicion due to lack of other signs and symptoms, such as swelling and arm disuse that typically are seen with other types of fractures. Given these minimal symptoms at the time of evaluation, it is estimated that over 20% of these fractures are initially missed. Radiographs of the forearm should include two views to fully assess for possible injury. Buckle fractures occur at the flare of the metaphysis. This area should be continuous and smooth. One way to better explain this is to visualize a marble rolling up the metaphysis; if it encounters any bumps on the way, that would be indicative of a fracture. It is important to closely examine the lateral film for similar smoothness, since some fractures will only involve the dorsal cortex, making it visible only on the lateral view (Figure 5.2). Buckle fractures are inherently stable and are not at risk for late displacement. Once the fracture is detected, management differs by local practice. Traditionally, these fractures are splinted with a follow-up casting. Alternatively, immediate casting can be performed. Immobilization typically lasts for 3 to 4 weeks. Recent studies have shown that patients treated with a removable forearm splint, worn for 2 to 4 weeks, had better physical

(a) (b)

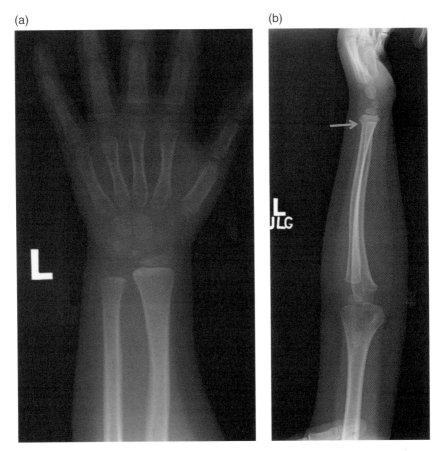

Figure 5.2 AP (a) and lateral (b) forearm of radial buckle fracture in a 3-year-old female. The AP view reveals no visible fracture. The lateral view has an abrupt change in angle of the dorsal cortex of the metaphysis, indicative of a buckle fracture.

function, less difficulty with daily activities, and less cost than traditional casting [3, 4].

> KEY FACT | **Over 20% of buckle fractures are missed on initial visit.**

Pitfall | **Failure to recognize a nursemaid's elbow**

Nursemaid's elbow is the most common joint injury in children. It happens when there is a sudden pull on the child's outstretched, pronated arm. This typically occurs in children younger than 6 years of age [5]. Over half of nursemaid's elbow cases will have a classic history of being pulled; the other half will describe a fall or an unclear history of trauma [6]. The pulling force dislocates the annular ligament that usually surrounds the head of the radius superiorly, trapping it between the radius and the capitellum of the humerus. To decrease discomfort, the child will minimize use of the hand by holding the arm close to the body, flexing at the elbow, and keeping the forearm pronated. Typically the child is apprehensive, but there is no true pain, swelling, or bruising about the elbow or forearm. Radiographs of the elbow are only necessary if there is a concerning history for fracture or any swelling, deformity, or bruising. When radiographs are obtained in nursemaid's elbow, they appear normal. There will be no visible dislocation since it is the

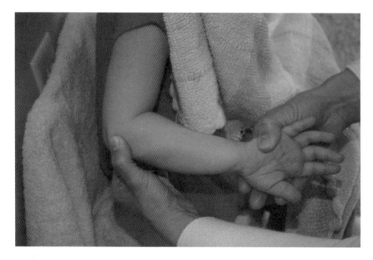

Figure 5.3 Hyperpronation method of nursemaid's elbow reduction With the child in the parent's lap, sit facing the child. Gently hold the child's elbow placing your thumb on the child's radial head then, with your other hand, grasp the child's pronated wrist. With moderate force and speed, hyperpronate the child's forearm, turning the child's thumb down and around until resistance is felt. A palpable pop should be felt about the elbow when reduction occurs.

annular ligament that is displaced, not the radial head. Frequently, the dislocation will be reduced during positioning for radiographs. To actively reduce the dislocation, two methods are suggested: hyperpronation (Figure 5.3) and supination/flexion. The hyperpronation method has been found to be less painful in children and more successful on the first attempt [7]. With the reduction maneuver, a palpable click is felt over the radial head. The child should start using the arm by 5 to 10 minutes after a successful reduction. Parental instruction on avoidance of picking the child up or swinging them by the arms is important to decrease recurrence. Even with this, nursemaid's elbow recurs in about 25% of children [8].

KEY FACT | **Nursemaid's elbow is a clinical diagnosis; x-rays are not necessary.**

Pitfall | **Failure to identify a posterior fat pad sign as an indicator of a supracondylar fracture**

Pediatric elbow injuries can be the most difficult in terms of fracture diagnosis, management, and the risk of complications. The normal anatomy of the pediatric elbow is challenging given that it is mainly a cartilaginous structure that ossifies with age. The six centers of ossification around the elbow progress chronologically (Figure 5.4).

One clue of an occult supracondylar fracture of the elbow is a posterior fat pad. A posterior fat pad of the distal humerus is indicative of a joint effusion or hemarthrosis (Figure 5.5). In the setting of trauma, a posterior fat pad is always pathologic and is pathognomonic for a type 1 supracondylar fracture. Another way to detect subtle misalignment of the elbow is to assess the capitellum for displacement by using the anterior humeral line. A line drawn down the anterior cortex of the humerus should transect the middle one-third of the capitellum. Usually, if there is displacement of the capitellum, this line will intersect more anteriorly on the capitellum. The radius should point directly toward and transect the center of the capitellum in all views. In uncertain cases, a comparison view should be obtained. If there is any concern for fracture, the limb should be splinted and follow-up arranged.

KEY FACT | **A subtle fracture of the elbow can be detected by looking for a posterior fat pad. A *posterior* fat pad of the elbow is always *pathologic*.**

Pitfall | **Missing a toddler's fracture in a young child refusing to bear weight and negative x-rays**

The young child with a limp or refusal to bear weight can pose a diagnostic challenge. One specific

(a)

(b)

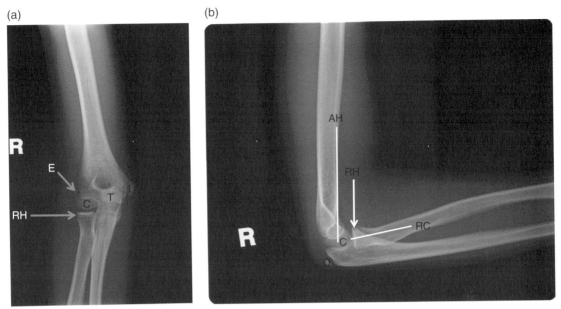

Figure 5.4 AP (a) and lateral (b) radiographs of normal right elbow in a 10-year-old female. Ossification centers of the pediatric elbow appear in order with approximate age; capitellum (C) (1 year of age), radial head (arrow RH) (3 years), internal condyle (I) (5 years), trochlea (T) (7 years), olecranon (O) (9 years), and external condyle (arrow E) (11 years). Note on the lateral view that the anterior humeral (AH) line transects the middle one-third of the capitellum and that the radio-capitellar (RC) line intersects with the middle of the capitellum.

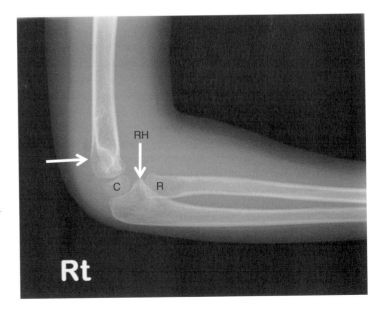

Figure 5.5 Lateral elbow radiograph at 4 years of age. Note posterior fat pad sign (arrow), indicative of occult supracondylar fracture. Capitellum (C) and radius (R), with a small developing radial head (RH arrow) are visible.

cause for refusal to bear weight in a child less than 3 years of age is a toddler's fracture. A toddler's fracture is defined as a spiral fracture of the middle or distal tibia that is minimally displaced or nondisplaced. Other considerations in the differential specific for this age are: foot foreign body, poorly fitting shoes, infection, and vaso-occlusive crisis. While most cases are associated with some sort of trauma, it is often relatively minor and may be dismissed by the parent or caregiver as trivial. If a mechanism is known, a torsional or rotational component is common. Planting of the foot and twisting of the leg or catching of the foot or leg in between the slats of a crib are frequent scenarios for toddler's fracture.

The clinical examination of a child that refuses to walk should include careful inspection of the thigh, leg, and foot and full range of motion of the hip, knee, and ankle. The most consistent clinical findings in children with toddler's fractures are the inability to bear weight and possibly focal bony tenderness. It is uncommon to find localized swelling or warmth. In fact, most children are quite happy as long as they are not made to put any weight on the affected extremity. The examiner may be able to elicit pain by placing an axial load on the tibia by compressing the foot toward the knee, or by creating a torsional force on the tibia by stabilizing the knee and rotating the foot. The ability to bear weight and take steps significantly decreases the likelihood of the presence of a toddler's fracture [9].

Radiographs of children with suspected toddler's fracture can be limited initially to an AP and lateral of the tibia and fibula. The AP radiograph is the most likely to reveal the hairline spiral fracture. If these are negative, additional oblique views can increase the likelihood of detection in some cases. Negative radiographs do not rule out this diagnosis. In one study, up to 41% of confirmed cases of toddler's fracture on follow up had negative radiographs on initial evaluation [9].

A presumptive diagnosis of toddler's fracture should be made in a young child with a history of acute injury, refusal to walk, and absence of signs or symptoms of infection. Treatment of the child with a suspected toddler's fracture should include immobilization in a long leg cast for comfort, to prevent displacement, and to promote healing. Follow up radiographs at 10–14 days out of the cast will often show periosteal new bone formation, confirming the diagnosis (Figure 5.6).

> **KEY FACT** | Over 40% of children with toddler's fracture will have negative initial radiographs. If clinical suspicion is high for toddler's fracture, the child should be placed in a long leg cast and have repeat radiographs performed in 2 weeks.

Pitfall | Not considering hip pathology when a young adolescent complains of distal thigh or knee pain

Slipped capital femoral epiphysis (SCFE) is a frequently missed, time-sensitive pediatric orthopedic problem. Delay in diagnosis may lead directly to worsening slippage, need for more aggressive surgery, and possible chronic hip arthritis. SCFE occurs at the proximal growth plate of the femur. The metaphysis of the femoral neck slips anteriorly and superiorly in relationship to the femoral head or epiphysis. The femoral head stays in the acetabulum due to the ligamentum teres. The majority of patients will present with a limp and pain in the hip, groin, or proximal thigh. Frequently, the pain is chronic, but acute slippage can occur with minor trauma. About 15% of children will only have knee or distal thigh pain at presentation of SCFE [10]. Also, within the differential diagnosis of hip pain is Legg–Calve Perthes disease (idiopathic osteonecrosis of the femoral head) and apophyseal avulsion fracture of the hip. The typical patient with SCFE will be an obese adolescent male that is going through a growth spurt. On examination, there is likely decreased range of hip motion, particularly with internal rotation. With hip flexion, frequently there will be obligate external rotation. Diagnosis is made on the AP and frog-leg lateral radiographs of both hips (Figure 5.7). A single AP view of the hips (Figure 5.7(a)) would miss approximately one-third of the SCFE cases. Bilateral hip involvement occurs in 20 to 40% of patients. The AP view will show widening or blurring (Bloomberg's sign) of the proximal femoral growth plate (Figure 5.7(b)).

(a) (b)

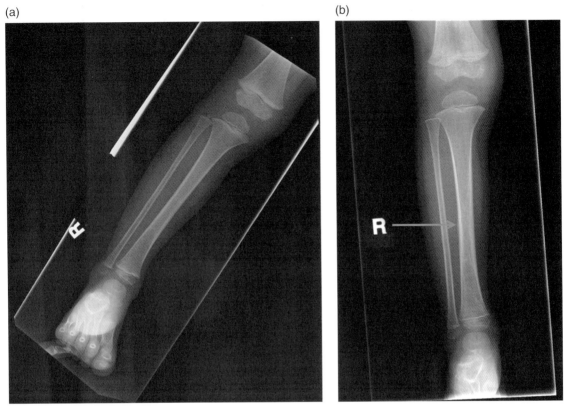

Figure 5.6 AP of tibia/fibula in a 2-year-old male. (a) Initial radiograph reveals no visible fracture. (b) Follow-up films at 2 weeks, reveals periosteal reaction and callus formation (arrow), confirming the diagnosis of a toddler's fracture.

(a) (b)

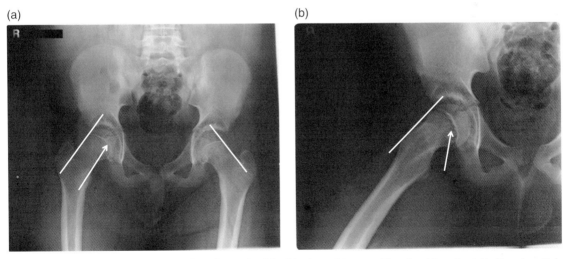

Figure 5.7 AP (a) and frog-leg lateral (b) radiograph of the hips in an 11-year-old male with early right slipped capital femoral epiphysis. Klein's line is drawn bilaterally; note that it does not intersect the femoral head on the right side. Note the blurring of the growth plate (arrow) (Bloomberg's sign).

The frog-leg lateral view is the best to appreciate displacement of the head of the femur. A line drawn along the superior aspect of femoral neck (Klein's line) should intersect with the lateral portion of the head of the femur. If a slip has occurred, Klein's line will not touch the head of the femur. A 2-millimeter or greater difference in distance of Klein's line from unaffected side to affected side improves the sensitivity of this measure (modified Klein's line). In severe slips, the head of the femur can take on an appearance analogous to a scoop of ice cream that has fallen off the cone. Once a SCFE has been diagnosed, the child should not bear any weight on that hip. Immediate orthopedic referral is necessary for surgical stabilization and prevention of further slippage.

> KEY FACT | **A frog-leg view of the hip should be ordered in addition to an AP view to diagnose SCFE.**

Pitfall | **Failure to consider septic arthritis in a young child with fever and a limp**

A septic joint requires rapid identification and treatment to avoid severe and permanent damage. Septic arthritis (SA) predominately occurs in the lower extremities. One must be diligent when a young child presents with fever and limp or refusal to walk. If the child appears ill with fever and has a warm, erythematous, painful joint, referral should immediately be made to an emergency department (ED) ideally with pediatric orthopedic services. However, in the child with fever and limp who does *not* appear ill, one must be thorough to evaluate for early SA. The hip joint has the greatest risk for long-term complications from SA. Early SA of the hip must be differentiated from transient synovitis (TS). TS is a reactive arthritis of the joint and is generally a diagnosis of exclusion. In both SA and TS, the position of comfort is with the hip flexed, abducted, and externally rotated. On examination, the child will have pain with hip range of motion, particularly with internal rotation. Anterior–posterior (AP) and frog-leg lateral radiographs of both hips should be obtained to exclude any bony abnormality. A subtle joint effusion may be appreciated on plain films in both SA and TS. Laboratory

> **Box 5.1** Kocher criteria for septic arthritis of the hip
>
> History of fever >38.5 °C (101.3 °F)
>
> Nonweight bearing
>
> ESR >40 mm/h
>
> WBC >12,000 cells/mm³
>
> If none of above criteria, the risk of septic hip is 2%
>
> | | |
> |---|---|
> | If one criteria | 10% |
> | If two criteria | 35% |
> | If three criteria | 73% |
> | If four criteria | 93% |
>
> Data from Kocher *et al.* [12]

evaluation is often necessary to stratify the patient for the likelihood of SA. The peripheral white blood cell count is normal in 80% of children with SA of the hip [11]. The Kocher criteria have been developed to help diagnose SA of the hip (Box 5.1) [12, 13]. In addition to the Kocher criteria, a C-reactive protein level less than 1 mg/dL is a strong negative predictor of SA [14]. Despite these predictors, a septic joint can often be a difficult diagnosis. In the authors' experience, many children with TS will respond well to ibuprofen, but this does not rule out SA. Because the diagnosis is crucial yet difficult to make, when in doubt, consider referral to the ED unless there is a structure that allows close follow-up and timely consultations.

> KEY FACT | **The peripheral white blood cell count is normal in 80% of children with SA of the hip.**

Pitfall | **Failing to recognize a fracture commonly associated with child abuse**

The true frequency of fractures related to child abuse is unknown. Estimates suggest that nearly 55% of abused children sustain a fracture at some point in time – second only to soft tissue injuries. It is clear is that many of these injuries go unrecognized, even when they present to healthcare providers. In a review of known abusive fractures, over 20% of children had at least one previous healthcare visit where the fracture was not recognized as abuse [15]. Young children and developmentally delayed children are at the highest risk for abuse.

The first step to detecting possible child abuse is being open to the possibility of its existence. Worrisome signs that a fracture is secondary to abuse include: a delayed presentation to care; inconsistent history; mechanism of injury described that is unlikely to result in the identified injury; multiple fractures; fractures in various stages of healing; and a large amount of callus around a healing fracture possibly due to improper immobilization. Once suspicion is present for abuse, a clinician should initiate the reporting and documentation process. Reporting requirements and procedures are specific to your practice location. The burden of proof does not rest on the shoulders of the clinician, but information gathered early in the evaluation may be critically valuable to social services and child protection agencies. The American Academy of Pediatrics Committee on Child Abuse and Neglect has issued a clinical report detailing the recommended evaluation of suspected child physical abuse [16]. Photo documentation of any cutaneous findings is important for future interpretation by a forensic expert. A complete skeletal survey should be considered mandatory for children less than 2 years of age and may be useful in developmentally disabled children up to 5 years of age who may not be able to provide a history. It is recommended that these radiographs be interpreted by a pediatric radiologist; consequently referral from the urgent care setting is often necessary. Infants should undergo retinal examination, by an ophthalmologist, as well as computed tomography (CT) of the head. Liver and pancreatic enzyme testing should be performed to evaluate for any potential intra-abdominal injuries. If any abnormalities are detected on physical examination or labs, CT of the abdomen and pelvis should be performed.

While there is no fracture that is truly pathognomonic, certain fracture patterns raise the suspicion for inflicted injury. It has been reported that up to 80% of all femur fractures in infants and 40% of all femur fractures in children are the result of abuse (Figure 5.8) [17]. A much higher percentage of femur fractures in nonambulatory children is associated with abuse (42% nonambulatory versus 2.6% of ambulatory) [16]. Contrary to common belief, one cannot rely on the type of femur fracture (i.e. spiral, oblique, or transverse) as a way to differentiate accidental from inflicted injury. Over half of children less than 3 years of age with humeral shaft fractures are likely to have been abused [17]. In contrast, supracondylar humeral fractures are almost always the result of accidents.

Skull fractures often raise suspicion for abuse. In children less than 3 years of age, skull fractures are the most common fracture seen in both abusive and nonabusive trauma. Thirty percent of skull fractures in infants and toddlers are the result of abuse [17]. The type of skull fracture is important. While simple linear skull fractures can be sustained from short falls (< 3 ft), multiple, comminuted or diastatic skull fractures described as the result of minor trauma are worrisome for abusive mechanism.

Rib fractures and metaphyseal fractures (i.e. corner fractures or bucket handle fractures) are the most highly suspicious fractures for abuse. Young children's ribs are quite flexible and therefore difficult to fracture in the absence of extreme force. The probability that a rib fracture is due to abuse is estimated to be over 70% [17]. The corner fracture of the distal femur, tibia, and proximal humerus are often due to traction or twisting of the extremity. These can produce minimal pain or deformity and heal without difficulty and thus may be easy to miss. Detection early in the injury can be challenging, and sometimes the fracture only becomes readily apparent on follow up x-rays when callous formation highlights the injury. In addition, the angle of the x-ray may change the appearance of the fracture. Tangential views will show triangular fracture fragments (corner fracture) whereas the oblique views may show a curvilinear appearance (bucket handle fracture).

Sternum, scapular and spine fractures are uncommon in children. Injury to these bones requires significant force, such as a from a motor vehicle accident. The absence of a clear history of such a mechanism should raise a clinician's concern.

> KEY FACT | **While there is no one fracture type that is truly pathognomonic for abuse, one must have a high index of suspicion for abuse when a young child presents with a femur or mid-shaft humerus fracture.**

(a) (b)

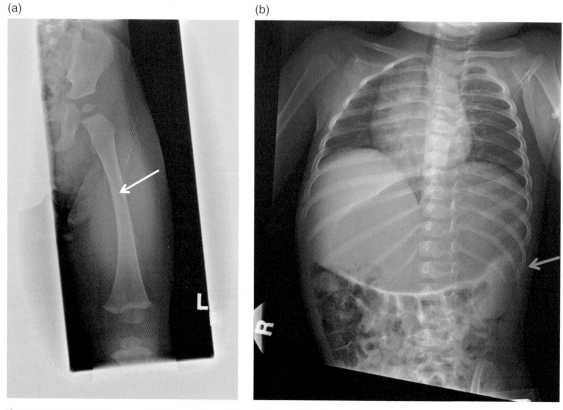

Figure 5.8 AP of left femur and oblique chest radiographs revealing femur fracture, and left lateral rib fracture in a 17-month-old infant. (a) Note the nondisplaced oblique fracture of the left femur. (b) Left lateral rib fracture shows callus formation from a healing previous fracture.

Pearls for improving patient outcomes

• Children with open growth plates are more likely to fracture through the growth plate than sustain a sprain.

• Many buckle fractures of the forearm will only be visible on the lateral film.

• Nurse maid's elbow can be diagnosed clinically. If the typical history of being pulled with an outstretched hand, without any other trauma is present a hyperpronation maneuver may be performed without radiographs.

• The presence of a posterior fat pad in the setting of traumatic injury to the elbow with otherwise normal radiographs is highly suggestive of occult fracture.

• Normal x-rays are common in toddler's fracture. Immobilization of the extremity should be based on clinical suspicion.

• A normal white count does not rule out the possibility of septic arthritis.

• Children frequently complain of knee pain, when in reality it is the hip that is the cause of the pathology.

• Child abuse should always be a consideration when a child has a fracture or bruising in an infant. Rib, metaphyseal fractures, midshaft humeral and femur fractures in infant and non-ambulatory toddlers are high risk for abuse.

References

1 Mann DC, Rajmaira S. Distribution of physeal and nonphyseal fractures in 2,650 long-bone fractures in children aged 0–16 years. *J Pediatr Orthop* 1990; **10**(6): 713–716.

2 Salter R, Harris W. Injuries involving the epiphyseal plate. *J Bone Joint Surg* 1963; **45A**: 587–622.

3 Plint AC, Perry JJ, Correll R, Gaboury I, Lawton L. A Randomized, Controlled Trial of Removable Splinting Versus Casting for Wrist Buckle Fractures in Children. *Pediatrics* 2006 March 1; **117**(3): 691–697.

4 Firmin F, Crouch R. Splinting versus casting of "torus" fractures to the distal radius in the paediatric patient presenting at the emergency department (ED): A literature review. *Inter Emerg Nurs* 2009; **17**(3): 173–178.

5 Schutzman SA, Teach S. Upper-Extremity Impairment in Young Children. *Ann Emerg Med* 1995; **26**(4): 474–479.

6 Schunk J. Radial head subluxation: epidemiology and treatment of 87 episodes. *Ann Emerg Med* 1990; **19**(9): 19–23.

7 Macias C, Bothner J, Wiebe R. A Comparison of Supination/Flexion to Hyperpronation in the Reduction of Radial Head Subluxations. *Pediatrics* 1998; **102**(e10).

8 Teach, Schutzman. Prospective study of recurrent radial head subluxation. *Arch Pediatr Adolesc Med* 1996; **150**(2): 164–166.

9 Halsey M, Finzel K, Carrion W, *et al.* Toddler's Fracture: Presumptive Diagnosis and Treatment. *J Pediatr Orthop* 2001; **21**(2): 152–156.

10 Matava M, Patton C, Luhmann S, *et al.* Knee pain as the initial symptom of slipped capital femoral epiphysis: an analysis of initial presentation and treatment. *J Pediatr Orthop* 1999; **19**(4): 455–460.

11 Laine JC, Kaiser SP, Diab M. High-risk pediatric orthopedic pitfalls. *Emerg Med Clin North Am* 2010; **28**(1): 85–102.

12 Kocher M, Zurakowski D, Kasser J. Differentiating Between Septic Arthritis and Transient Synovitis of the Hip in Children: An Evidence-Based Clinical Prediction Algorithm. *J Bone Joint Surg Am* 1999 Dec. 1, 1999; **81**(12): 1662–1670.

13 Kocher MS, Mandiga R, Zurakowski D, *et al.* Validation of a Clinical Prediction Rule for the Differentiation Between Septic Arthritis and Transient Synovitis of the Hip in Children. *J Bone Joint Surg, Am Vol* 2004 Aug; **86**(8): 1629–1635.

14 Caird MS, Flynn JM, Leung YL, *et al.* Factors distinguishing septic arthritis from transient synovitis of the hip in children. A prospective study. *J Bone Joint Surg, Am Vol* 2006 June; **88**(6): 1251–1257.

15 Ravichandiran N, Schuh S, Bejuk M, *et al.* Delayed identification of pediatric abuse-related fractures. *Pediatrics* 2010; **125**(1): 60–66.

16 Kellogg N, Committee on Child Abuse and Neglect. Evaluation of Suspected Child Physical Abuse. *Pediatrics* 2007 June; **119**(6): 1232–1241.

17 Kemp AM, Dunstan F, Harrison S, *et al.* Patterns of skeletal fractures in child abuse: systematic review. *BMJ* 2008; **337**: a1518.

CHAPTER 6
Pitfalls of Wound Management

Michael K. Abraham[1] and Hyung T. Kim[2]

[1] Department of Emergency Medicine, University of Maryland School of Medicine, Baltimore, MD, USA

[2] Department of Emergency Medicine, University of Southern California, Los Angeles County Hospital, Los Angeles, CA, USA

Introduction

A discussion of wound care is rarely ground-breaking; however, the use of older methods for cleaning and treating wounds can lead to poor outcomes and significant patient morbidity. This is even more apparent when the practitioner does not have access to a plethora of specialists to assist with the evaluation and management. Wound care constitutes a large part of the care provided in any acute care facility. Mainly due to the sheer volume of patients with injuries requiring wound care, this topic generates a major amount of litigation. It is estimated that between 5% and 20% of all malpractice claims, and more than 10% of all malpractice dollars are spent on issues associated with wound care [1].

The main aspects of wound care that interest patients are cosmetic and functional outcomes, pain relief and infection control. The key to understanding wound care is realizing that the repair is only the beginning of the treatment. Successful outcomes depend on both the provider and the patient. If the practitioner closes the wound poorly, healing will be less than optimal from the outset. The same is also true if the patient does not comply with post-treatment instructions; where the outcome, despite the practitioner's meticulous closure, will be less than optimal.

Wound preparation

Pitfall | **Failure to properly prepare the wound before repair**

Although there are many factors that influence wound healing, no single action is of more importance than proper wound preparation. Prior to closure, proper preparation of the wound can prevent a significant amount of morbidity, namely from infection, that is associated with traumatic wounds. In general, the most important aspects of traumatic wound preparation are appropriate irrigation and debridement of necrotic tissue in the wound. When approaching a traumatic wound the practitioner should first focus on irrigation. The amount of irrigation necessary for the wound is directly related to the expected amount of contamination. In many cases, highly contaminated wounds can require ten times more irrigation than clean injuries. Another aspect that needs to be taken into consideration is the area where the laceration occurs. Highly vascular areas, for example the face or scalp, require less irrigation to prevent infections. Studies have shown no difference in the rates of infection in clean facial and scalp wounds regardless of irrigation [2]. In contrast, irrigation of a foot wound in a diabetic patient necessitates profuse irrigation. The next step in preparing the wound for closure is determining which irrigation solution to use and how it should be applied. Irrigation should be just that,

Urgent Care Emergencies: Avoiding the Pitfalls and Improving the Outcomes, First Edition.
Edited by Deepi G. Goyal and Amal Mattu.

© 2012 John Wiley & Sons, Ltd. Published 2012 by John Wiley & Sons, Ltd.

irrigation and not soaking. Soaking wounds in iodine solution has shown to be ineffective in preventing, and may even promote infections [3]. Although most practitioners believe that the use of sterile solutions is mandatory, irrigation with tap water is equally effective for uncomplicated wounds [4, 5].

> KEY FACT | **Soaking wounds in iodine solution has shown to be ineffective in preventing, and may even promote infections.**

What seems to be most important is the amount and pressure with which the wound is irrigated. The most effective technique is to irrigate at pressures of 5 to 8 psi. To do this use a 20- to 60-mL syringe with a 19 to 20 gauge needle or angiocath [4]. Caution must be used as overzealous irrigation at pressures higher than necessary may result in further damage to the tissue. Take care not to apply too much pressure to areas with delicate microvasculature, like the eye and ear. Over-aggressive irrigation in these areas can separate the overlying tissue from the cartilage and cause necrosis [6]. A volume of 50 to 100 mL per centimeter of wound is a good place to begin. The use of tissue toxic solutions should be avoided. These include provodine–iodine solutions and hydrogen peroxide. These solutions can devitalize the healthy tissue and provide a medium for bacteria to flourish, thus impairing wound healing [7]. There is some evidence to suggest that the use of a 1% provodine–iodine solution in infection-prone wounds is beneficial [8, 9]. This, however, is controversial because this antiseptic, especially in higher concentration, impairs wound healing. Its use may be justified when there are no alternatives, but everyone has access to tap water.

> KEY FACT | **Wounds should be irrigated with 50–100 mL per centimeter.**

Foreign bodies

Pitfall | **Failure to inform the patient about the possibility of a foreign body**

On the initial evaluation of a patient one of the key aspects of the history that must be obtained by the practitioner is the possibility of the presence of a foreign body. There are a few aspects of the history that should alert the practitioner to be more aggressive in the evaluation for a foreign body. These include injuries caused by glass, foreign body sensation, or persistent pain and drainage [10]. After a thorough history, the physical examination can help to elucidate, but not eliminate, the possibility of a retained foreign body. The most ideal situation would be to examine all wounds in the absence of blood and through the entire length of the wound. This would seem to eliminate any chance of a foreign body; however, even with direct visualization of the base of the wound there remains an almost 20% chance of a retained foreign body [1].

Any injury that was caused by or affected by glass should be evaluated with an imaging modality, since the most likely retained foreign body is glass. In the past, the use of plain films was the only way to evaluate for foreign bodies. Although the use of plain radiography does further reduce the possibility of a retained foreign body, it does have some limitations. Wounds that retain vegetative matter, for example wood or thorns, may not have any noticeable abnormality on films. It must also be considered that some forms of plastic are radiolucent and will be very difficult or impossible to visualize. The unfortunate paradox is that wounds caused by these objects have a higher likelihood of becoming infected, which places the practitioner in a difficult situation. The use of multiple views and markers (e.g. paper clips) can be helpful in determining the location of foreign bodies in three dimensions when using plain films.

> KEY FACT | **Even with direct visualization of the base of the entire wound, there remains up to a 20% chance of a retained foreign body.**

If your facility is fortunate enough to have other imaging modalities, these can be extremely useful in the detection of foreign bodies. Most hospital-based facilities will have computed tomography (CT) scanning and ultrasound services, in addition to plain films. CT scanning has gained popularity since it compensates for many of the inadequacies of plain radiography. CT scanning has two main advantages to plain films in that it is 100 times more sensitive for the detection of a foreign body and it also allows for a three-dimensional determination of the object [11]. The use of ultrasound to visualize retained objects has a unique benefit when compared to other modalities in that it allows for 'real time' visualization. In essence, you can search for the object with forceps or a needle and determine your location when compared with the object [12]. Both CT scanning and ultrasound use may not be readily available and the patient may ultimately need referral for further management.

One important fact to remember is that injuries are not the only causes of retained foreign bodies. Occasionally the repair of a wound can necessitate the use of deep sutures to facilitate closing. These deep sutures are, in essence, foreign bodies and will provoke an immune response. Deep sutures should only be used when they are absolutely necessary and should be limited to areas that are less likely to become infected.

Plantar wounds

Pitfall | **Failure to appreciate the high-risk nature of plantar puncture wounds**

Patients presenting with plantar wounds provide a difficult situation for the acute care practitioner. Patients do not always present immediately after the injury since bleeding is not usually a major concern from these injuries. In addition to the delayed time from the injury to presentation there are other factors that influence the rates of infection. The three main factors that influence the propensity for plantar wounds to become infected are the mechanism of injury, the inherently contaminated area of the foot, and the structural anatomy. A particular concern for the practitioner is the fact that most plantar wounds are punctures. Unlike a laceration that is formed by a sweeping motion of a sharp object, a puncture wound is formed by pushing perpendicular to the epidermis. This force acts to push foreign bodies into the wound and trap them there as the object is removed. In addition, the skin

may actually close at the surface depending on the size of the object causing the injury, effectively sealing the contaminants into the wound. While the mechanism is important to understand the risk of infection, it is also imperative to understand the bacterial flora present in the plantar area, and how this can change with different footwear. As we walk, our feet are in constant contact with the surrounding environment. This interaction provides countless opportunities for wounds to occur on the plantar surface. Overall Gram-positive bacteria are the most common bacteria found in plantar wound infections; however, when the injury involves rubber-soled shoes *Pseudomonas* infection must be considered [10]. Therefore, when the wound occurs through rubber-soled shoes, the use of ciprofloxacin should be considered as first-line therapy.

> KEY FACT | **When the wound occurs through rubber-soled shoes, the use of ciprofloxacin should be considered as first-line therapy.**

The final characteristic of plantar wounds that contributes to their morbidity is the structural anatomy of the foot. The proximity of the skin to important structures such as joints, in conjunction with the force exerted onto the foot from the weight of the individual contributes to high rates of osteomyelitis. The fact that the feet, as body parts, are the farthest from the central circulation can contribute to the increased propensity for infection. Treatment for plantar punctures is generally the same for all other types of wounds. There should be a thorough search for retained foreign bodies which can include plain radiographs or referral for more sensitive tests. Although the wound should be cleansed using high pressure (5–8 psi) with a nontoxic solution, one cannot simply place the needle into the puncture wound as this may force contaminants into the wound. If the wound is small and prevents adequate irrigation, the puncture wound can be converted into a laceration to aid in proper irrigation. Wounds that are grossly infected can be "cored out," leaving a large area for drainage of the infection [13]. Finally, as mentioned above, the judicious use of antibiotics is indicated for these wounds, keeping in mind the prevailing organisms.

Wound care instructions

Pitfall | **Failure to provide appropriate wound care and follow up instructions**

One of the most important and often overlooked aspects of wound care is the post-discharge care set of instructions. The time spent with the practitioner is minuscule in comparison to the total time the wound needs to heal. Proper instructions can eliminate some of the long-term complications that are inherent with traumatic wounds. These instructions should be succinct, easily understandable, and most importantly provide the patient with reasonable expectations of the healing process. One of the main concerns for patients presenting for wound care is cosmesis, or the visual appearance of the healed wound [14]. It is important to explain the healing process of the wound, especially that all wounds leave scars caused by the healing process. Patients should also be recommended to avoid UV light exposure during the wound-healing process, as this may produce permanent hyperpigmentation of the wound.

In an effort to save time and promote understanding the instructions can be given twice, with the first being during the closure of the wound. The patient at this point is a captive audience and this allows the practitioner to have the patient's full attention. The second set of instructions comes prior to discharge with more formal written instructions that the patient can keep for future reference. The instructions should discuss cleaning, bandages, antibiotic ointments, and follow-up. Cleaning closed wounds is always advised. As discussed previously, harsh tissue toxic materials like hydrogen peroxide should not be used. The wounds can be cleansed with mild soap and water and then dried carefully, usually by patting dry. This can happen as early as 4 to 6 hours after closure. Drying the wound is an especially important point to convey since wounds that are excessively wet can cause the skin at the edges of the wound to degrade and ultimately cause dehiscence of the wound. The choice of bandage should be guided by the location of the wound. The bandage should protect the wound from contamination, trauma, and sunlight while allowing for proper environment for wound

healing. If the patient is expected to change the dressings, explicit instructions on dressing changes must be provided. The use of bacitracin is very common but current data suggests that it is a common cause of contact dermatitis and may impede wound healing [15]. Over-the-counter petroleum-based antibiotic ointments are effective and there is little to no disadvantage to their use [16]. The final aspect of the instructions should provide return instructions. Most wounds should be re-evaluated by a healthcare provider within 48 hours, although this is just a guideline and remains highly flexible and patient dependent. Highly contaminated wounds or bites may need to be examined within 24 hours. Conversely, clean wounds in a reliable patient may not need to be seen until the removal of sutures. The patient should be instructed to return at the first sign of infection, even if it is before the scheduled follow-up visit. Finally, the patient should be given clear instructions on when to have the sutures or staples removed.

Zipper injuries

Pitfall | **Failure to appropriately manage zipper injuries**

Although not very common, zipper injuries can be both emotionally and physically painful to the patient. Due to the anatomy of the region boys tend to be affected more frequently than girls. If the skin is entrapped within the sliding mechanism the extrication can be challenging. An acute care provider will be tempted to release the entrapped skin by forcibly unzipping. This procedure can result in repeated trauma and should be reserved as the last resort. The technique for extrication is based on the location of the skin in relation to the sliding mechanism. If the skin is entrapped between the teeth of the zipper, a provider can cut the cloth around the affected area and gently pull apart the teeth of the zipper (Figure 6.1). The most common method involves using wire or bone cutters to cut the median bar, separate the anterior and posterior faceplates and release the skin. The median bar may be quite strong and will require a considerable amount of force when

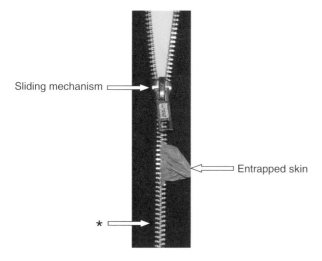

Sliding mechanism

Entrapped skin

*

Figure 6.1 Cut below the entrapped skin (*) and pull the teeth of the zipper apart to release it.

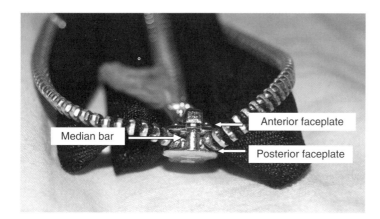

Anterior faceplate

Median bar

Posterior faceplate

Figure 6.2 Anatomy of zipper's sliding mechanism.

severing it. Another option is to soak the affected skin in mineral oil for approximately 15 minutes before gently pulling the skin away from the teeth [17].

Another reported mechanism for removing the faceplate is to insert a small flathead screwdriver between the faceplate and rotating toward the median bar to release the skin (Figure 6.2). There is no single superior method to treat a zipper injury [18]. Each case must be treated individually and the appropriate technique applied. Besides considering the suitable technique, the provider should not overlook the importance of analgesia and sedation, especially in pediatric patients. The weight of the pants can cause more pain and trauma, thus the provider must work swiftly to cut the clothes

around the injury to release tension and gain access to the area. Cases in younger children may require general anesthesia and possible circumcision. Emergent consultation is required in these cases.

Burn management

Pitfall | **Overlooking burns to high-risk areas**

Acute care providers regularly treat small and superficial burns. These wounds should be managed with careful cleaning using mild soap and water, topical antibiotics such as silver sulfadiazine and dry dressing [19]. Unfortunately, all burns are not as easily treated. Providers must be aware of the types of burns that may be at high risk for infection, disfigurement, and loss of function. For example, the treatment of facial burns requires special consideration. Although silver sulfadiazine is widely used for most burns, it should be avoided on the face due to its mild bleaching effect. Silver sulfadiazine should also be avoided in pregnant women and nursing mothers since it may cause kernicterus in infants. The use of bacitracin, even with its increased risk of contact dermatitis, is an excellent alternative in these cases. When the burn involves the eye, the provider needs to carefully assess the eye and surrounding structures. The injured area requires copious irrigation to remove debris and cool the surface of the cornea. Burns around the eyes and cornea are treated with topical ophthalmic antibiotic ointment and a generous application of artificial tears. Any burns to the eyelid should raise the alarm since they may result in permanent contractures and an inability to close the eyelid. Thus, patients with these burns should be referred to a burn center for further management.

> KEY FACT | Silver sulfadiazine should be avoided in pregnant women and nursing mothers since it may cause kernicterus in infants

Burns to the hands pose many challenges upon initial presentation. The provider must assess the vascular integrity as these injuries are at high risk for compartment syndrome. If there is concern for compromised blood flow to the hands and fingers, the patient should be referred promptly to a burn center for further management as an emergent escharotomy or fasciotomy may be required. The burnt hand should be splinted in a position of function and elevated to decrease edema. Each digit should be dressed separately to prevent adherence to one another. Early mobility and rehabilitation is often recommended to preserve function and decrease the risk of long-term contractures. Extensive burns to the face, hands, feet and perineum – as well as patients who meet the criteria for a major burn – should be transferred to a burn center [20].

In pediatric cases, child abuse should be considered whenever a toddler presents with delineated and symmetrical burns to the buttock or thighs, which are suggestive of scalding by immersion. A deep circular wound should raise suspicion of a cigarette burn. If there are any concerns, prompt referral to child protective services is warranted.

Depending on the location of your practice, sunburn may represent a large portion of your burnt patients. Luckily the short-term treatment of these injuries is mainly supportive. The key to proper sunburn treatment lies in the prevention of the injury with proper sun protection. The patient will present with erythema, warmth, tenderness, and even blistering if severe enough [21]. If the patient is presenting for treatment, analgesia with NSAIDS or acetaminophen is appropriate. The use of aloe and steroids, both systemic and topical, are controversial. These agents may help with symptoms but do not shorten recovery time, and the use of steroids can increase the risk of systemic infection in severe burns.

Pearls for improving patient outcomes

• The most important aspects of wound preparation are appropriate irrigation and debridement of necrotic tissue in the wound.
• Evaluate every wound for the presence of foreign bodies, and inform the patient about the possibility of their existence.
• Beware the high risk of infection in patients with plantar puncture wounds.
• Provide appropriate analgesia when treating patients with zipper injuries.
• Avoid the use of silver sulfadiazine on the face, in pregnant patients, and in nursing mothers.
• Maintain a low threshold for transferring patients with hand burns to burn centers.

References

1 Pfaff J, Moore G. ED wound management; identifying and reducing risk. *ED Legal Letter* 2005; **16**: 97–108.
2 Hollander JE, Singer AJ. Laceration management. *Ann Emerg Med* 1999; **34**: 356–367.

3 Chisholm CD. Wound evaluation and cleansing. *Emerg Med Clin North Am* 1992; **10**: 665–672.

4 Capellan O, Hollander JE. Management of lacerations in the emergency department. *Emerg Med Clin North Am* 2003; **21**: 205–231.

5 Bansal BC, Wiebe RA, Perkins SD, Abramo TJ. Tap water for irrigation of lacerations. *Am J Emerg Med* 2002; **20**: 469–472.

6 Brown DJ, Jaffe JE, Henson JK. Advanced laceration management. *Emerg Med Clin North Am* 2007; **25**: 83–99.

7 Oberg MS, Lindsey D. Do not put hydrogen peroxide or povidone iodine into wounds! *Am J Dis Child* 1987; **141**: 27–28.

8 Oberg MS. Povidone-iodine solutions in traumatic wound preparation. *Am J Emerg Med* 1987; **5**: 553–555.

9 Dire DJ, Welsh AP. A comparison of wound irrigation solutions used in the emergency department. *Ann Emerg Med* 1990; **19**: 704–708.

10 Moayedi S, Torres M. Wound care in emergency medicine. In: Mattu A, Goyal D (eds.), *Emergency Medicine. Avoiding the Pitfalls and Improving Outcomes*. Malden: Blackwell; 2007: pp. 72–78.

11 Bauer AR, Jr., Yutani D. Computed tomographic localization of wooden foreign bodies in children's extremities. *Arch Surg* 1983; **118**: 1084–1086.

12 Dean AJ, Gronczewski CA, Costantino TG. Technique for emergency medicine bedside ultrasound identification of a radiolucent foreign body. *J Emerg Med* 2003; **24**: 303–308.

13 Lammers RL. Principles of wound management. In: Roberts JR, Hedges JR (eds.), *Roberts: Clinical Procedures in Emergency Medicine* (5th edn.). Philadelphia: Saunders Elsevier; 2009: p. 565.

14 Singer AJ, Mach C, Thode HC,Jr., *et al*. JE. Patient priorities with traumatic lacerations. *Am J Emerg Med* 2000; **18**: 683–686.

15 Saik RP, Walz CA, Rhoads JE. Evaluation of a bacitracin-neomycin surgical skin preparation. *Am J Surg* 1971; **121**: 557–560.

16 Smack DP, Harrington AC, Dunn C, *et al*. Infection and allergy incidence in ambulatory surgery patients using white petrolatum vs bacitracin ointment. *A randomized controlled trial. JAMA* 1996; **276**: 972–977.

17 Kanegaye JT, Schonfeld N. Penile zipper entrapment: A simple and less threatening approach using mineral oil. *Pediatr Emerg Care* 1993; **9**: 90–91.

18 Inoue N, Crook SC, Yamamoto LG. Comparing 2 methods of emergent zipper release. *Am J Emerg Med* 2005; **23**: 480–482.

19 Singer AJ, Dagum AB. Current management of acute cutaneous wounds. *N Engl J Med* 2008; **359**: 1037–1046.

20 McKee DM. Acute management of burn injuries to the hand and upper extremity. *J Hand Surg Am* 2010; **35**: 1542–1544.

21 Lowe NJ. An overview of ultraviolet radiation, sunscreens, and photo-induced dermatoses. *Dermatol Clin* 2006; **24**: 9–17.

CHAPTER 7

Emergency Dermatology for the Acute Care Provider

Eric T. Boie[1] and Jennifer A. Lisowe[2]

[1] Department of Emergency Medicine, Mayo Clinic, Rochester, MN, USA

[2] Department of Dermatology, Mayo Clinic Health System, Rochester, MN, USA

Introduction

Dermatologic problems represent about 15–20% of visits to acute care settings [1]. While most dermatologic problems are benign, skin problems can represent cutaneous manifestations of severe underlying medical disease. Such entities require early recognition by the acute care provider to ensure prompt treatment in a setting matching the patient's acuity.

The primary objective of this chapter is to outline a rational approach to the patient who presents with a rash in an urgent care setting. Figure 7.1 outlines this in detail. Three questions will be central to this approach: (1) Does the patient with a rash have findings and features suggestive of serious systemic medical disease or toxicity (i.e. a dermatologic emergency)? (2) Does the patient have a common, clinically identifiable disease for which treatment can be initiated? (3) Does the patient have a problem for which corticosteroid therapy, topical or oral, will be beneficial? Using these questions the acute care provider can more efficiently, safely, and effectively manage patients who present with a rash.

Dermatologic emergencies

Pitfall | **Failure to recognize a rash as a manifestation of a life-threatening underlying condition, constituting a dermatologic emergency**

The first objective in evaluating any patient with a rash is to identify signs, symptoms, or clinical features that are suggestive of a life-threatening dermatologic emergency. These are detailed in Box 7.1. A full set of vital signs must be obtained on any patient presenting with a rash. Vital sign abnormalities, rashes with extensive blistering, skin sloughing, or mucosal involvement, and the presence of petechiae all increase the likelihood that the patient has a dermatologic emergency. Patients with dermatologic emergencies presenting to an urgent care setting will require prompt transfer to a higher level of care and early initiation of treatment to prevent morbidity and mortality. We will discuss five dermatologic emergencies in detail: Rocky Mountain Spotted Fever, meningococcemia, Steven-Johnson syndrome – toxic epidermal necrolysis, staphylococcal toxic shock syndrome, and necrotizing

Urgent Care Emergencies: Avoiding the Pitfalls and Improving the Outcomes, First Edition.
Edited by Deepi G. Goyal and Amal Mattu.
© 2012 John Wiley & Sons, Ltd. Published 2012 by John Wiley & Sons, Ltd.

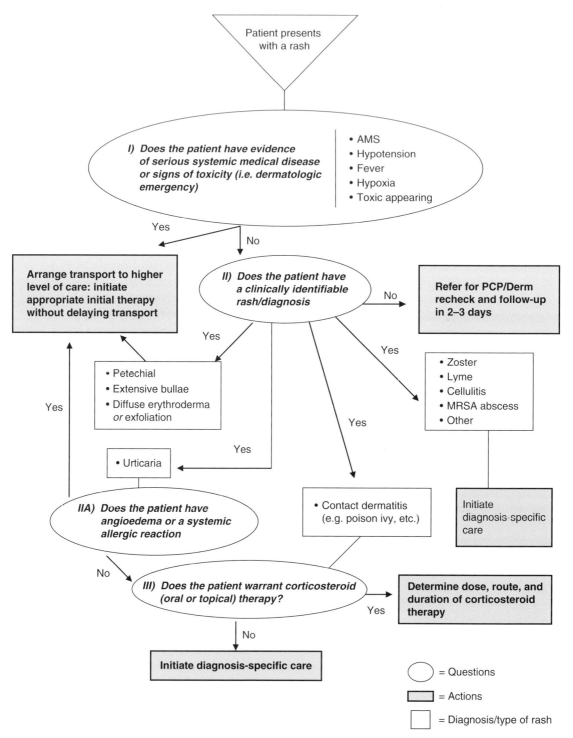

Figure 7.1 Approach to the patient who presents with a rash.

Box 7.1 Signs, symptoms, and clinical features suggestive of a dermatologic emergency

Hypotension

Tachycardia

Hypoxia

Fever > 38.9 °C (102 °F)

Pain out of proportion to clinical findings

Toxicity (ill-appearance)

Altered mental status

Dyspnea

Mucosal involvement (genital, oral, or conjunctival)

Extensive blistering, skin sloughing, or desquamation

Petechiae

fasciitis. These entities exemplify the findings and features suggestive of serious underlying disease in the patient presenting with a rash.

Pitfall | **Failure to identify a petechial rash**

Petechiae are small (1–2 mm) red or purple lesions which result from hemorrhages under the skin. They are usually flat and do not blanch when pressed upon. While petechial rashes may be benign secondary to trauma or viral infection, they are often seen in more serious conditions including Rocky Mountain Spotted Fever and meningococcemia. The acute care provider should assume a threatening cause of petechiae until proven otherwise.

Rocky Mountain Spotted Fever

Rocky Mountain Spotted Fever (RMSF is a tick-borne illness caused by *Rickettsia rickettsii*, a small Gram-negative bacterium. *Ixodidae* ticks are the natural hosts for this organism, consisting of the wood tick (*Dermacentor andersoni*) in western North America and the dog tick (*Dermacentor variabilis*) in eastern North America. Despite its name, most cases occur in the southern Atlantic and south central United States. Ninety percent of cases occur between April and September [2]. People with the highest likelihood of exposure to ticks are at the

greatest risk. Classic clinical presentation is fever, headache, and rash in a person with a history of tick exposure. Severe abdominal pain is common in children. The rash usually appears 2 to 5 days after the onset of fever in 80–90% of patients [3]. It begins around the wrists and ankles as small, blanching nonpruritic macules that progress to nonblanching petechial lesions involving palms, soles, trunk, and extremities with the face usually spared. Diagnosing RMSF is challenging; 60–75% of patients with this condition are given an alternate diagnosis at the initial physician visit [4]. Doxycycline 100 mg orally BID for 7 to 10 days is first-line therapy. If index of suspicion for RMSF is high, the patient should be transferred as complications include shock, acute renal failure, seizures, coma, and hepatic failure.

> KEY FACT | **Rocky Mountain Spotted Fever is associated with a mortality of 3–7% among treated patients and a 30–70% mortality among those not treated promptly or adequately.**

Meningococcemia

Neisseria meningitides, a Gram-negative diplococcus bacterium, is a leading cause of septicemia and meningitis among small children and young adults in North America and is associated with high mortality [5]. The clinical presentation of invasive meningococcal disease is variable and not necessarily associated with meningitis. Classically, the patient presents with an upper respiratory infection prodrome followed by abrupt onset of flu-like symptoms including fever, malaise, lethargy, mental status changes, and a rash [6]. The rash is the pathognomonic feature of meningococcemia and must be promptly identified by the acute care provider. The rash develops later in the disease course, beginning as a painful maculopapular rash. In 50–60% of cases it evolves into a petechial rash starting on the wrists, ankles, and axillae, and spreading to the trunk and extremities [7]. Head, palms, and soles are often spared. Petechiae then progress to stellate purpura with the characteristic central gunmetal-gray hue. If it is unrecognized or untreated, the disease can rapidly progress to shock, disseminated intravascular coagulation, acute renal failure, and death. Early recognition, prompt antibiotic administration using either IV penicillin G or ceftriaxone, and transfer to a facility with intensive care capabilities, are critical.

Pitfall | Failure to examine a patient with a rash for mucosal involvement

Stevens-Johnson Syndrome (SJS) and Toxic Epidermal Necrolysis (TEN) are conditions that represent a spectrum of drug-induced or idiopathic mucocutaneous reaction patterns. Roughly 50% of SJS and 80–90% of TEN patients are drug-induced with the most commonly implicated agents being sulfa drugs, anticonvulsants, and NSAIDS [1, 8]. Both are characterized by viral prodrome (fever, malaise, headache, cough) followed by development of a macular exanthema which begins centrally then spreads to the extremities. Atypical target lesions with central dusky purpura can be seen [9]. The exanthem eventually becomes confluent, and then converts to blistering with dermal–epidermal dissociation and sloughing. This denudation which occurs with shear stress is termed "a positive Nikolsky's sign."

> KEY FACT | The clinical hallmark of SJS and TEN is mucous membrane involvement with erythema and erosions of oral, genital, and ocular mucosa.

TEN and SJS are differentiated by percent body surface area (BSA) that is involved with <10% defined as SJS, 5–30% BSA defined as SJS/TEN, and >30% defined as TEN [9]. Epithelial sloughing results in susceptibility to bacterial infection, septicemia, and significant fluid loss. Mortality ranges from 5% in SJS to 30% in TEN [1]. These patients will need supportive care which includes intravenous fluids, corticosteroids, antimicrobials, and potentially burn-unit care if there is extensive body surface involved.

Pitfall | Failure to elicit a history of tampon use in a woman presenting with a diffuse rash and fever

Staphylococcal toxic shock syndrome (STSS) is a multisystem, fulminant illness induced by toxins produced by various strains of *Staphylococcus aureus*

bacteria. It is most often observed in menstruating women using highly absorbant tampons or in patients with nasal packing [1]. After a 2- to 3-day prodrome of malaise, patients typically present with fever, chills, nausea, abdominal pain, and hypotension. The rash of STSS typically develops in the first 48 hours of the illness. It is erythematous, nonpruritic, blanching, maculopapular or petechial and may have a "sandpaper" quality on palpation. Desquamation of the skin generally occurs 1 to 2 weeks following the onset of symptoms [10]. Six criteria must be met for the diagnosis of STSS: (1) fever >/= 38.9; (2) diffuse macular erythema; (3) desquamation at 1–2 weeks; (4) hypotension or orthostatic syncope; (5) evidence for the absence of other illness, i.e. sepsis; and (6) clinical or laboratory findings in at least three other organ systems: gastrointestinal, renal, hematologic, neurologic, hepatic, musculoskeletal, or mucosal membrane. Treatment is prompt removal of inciting factor (i.e. tampon), fluid resuscitation, and intravenous beta-lactamase-resistant, antistaphylococcal antibiotics.

Pitfall | Failure to recognize pain out of proportion to physical findings, thereby errantly diagnosing necrotizing fasciitis as simple cellulitis

Necrotizing fasciitis is defined as any necrotizing soft-tissue infection rapidly spreading along fascial planes, with or without overlying cellulitis [11]. Risk factors for developing necrotizing fasciitis include diabetes, severe peripheral vascular disease, alcohol or injection drug use, malnutrition, and obesity. Necrotizing fasciitis can be caused by multiple synergistic bacteria (Type I) or a single organism (Type II) such as group-A beta-hemolytic streptococcus. The most common sites are the abdomen, lower extremities, and perineum (Fournier's Gangrene). Initially patients develop tender, warm, edematous skin which then becomes dusky blue and insensate [10]. Hemorrhagic bullae then develop – the presence of which strongly signals necrotizing fasciitis [9]. Pain out of proportion to clinical examination findings, as well as the presence of crepitus (35% of cases), differentiate necrotizing fasciitis from simple cellulitis [12]. Such pain should not be attributed to drug or attention-seeking behavior. While broad spectrum antibiotic therapy is indicated, surgical debridement is the mainstay of treatment.

> KEY FACT | **Necrotizing fasciitis has a mortality rate of 25% which increases to 70% in those patients who develop sepsis [13].**

Pitfall | **Failure to evaluate for angiodema or anaphylaxis in a patient with acute urticaria**

Urticaria is a common entity with 20% of the population experiencing hives, angioedema, or both at some point in their life [14]. Urticaria universally has wheals. Wheals are defined by three features: (1) central swelling of various sizes, with or without surrounding erythema; (2) pruritus or occasional burning sensations; and (3) the skin returning to normal appearance, usually within 1–24 hours [15]. The provider must entertain other diagnoses that can mimic urticaria such as exanthems, photosensitivity reactions, and drug hypersensitivities, particularly if individual wheals are not fleeting in less than 24 hours. While individual wheals are fleeting, acute urticaria itself can last up to 6 weeks.

Evaluation of the patient with acute urticaria should begin with a quick assessment of the patient's vital signs and respiratory status for instability, suggesting angioedema or a generalized anaphylactic reaction. Angioedema can be associated with urticaria in 50% of cases [1]. Angioedema is a distinctive reaction pattern characterized by well-circumscribed areas of edema caused by increased vascular permeability, typically involving the face and upper respiratory tract. Involvement of the upper airway can be fatal as edema can progress to airway obstruction. The airway should be promptly secured in any patient with significant upper airway angioedema (lips, tongue, uvula, etc.). Treatment includes histamine blockers, steroids, and epinephrine if there is pending airway compromise. Patients with anaphylactic reaction (urticaria, wheezing, hypotension, hypoxia) should likewise be treated with antihistamines, corticosteroids, and epinephrine and transferred.

If the patient is stable, the medical history and physical examination are the best methods of

---

> **Box 7.2** Common causes of acute urticaria
>
> Infections
> - Viral (rhinovirus, rotavirus hepatitis A, B, C, Ebstein–Barr virus, herpes virus)
> - Bacterial (streptococcal, mycoplasma)
>
> Foods, preservatives, dyes
>
> Medications, vitamins, supplements
>
> Transfusions
>
> Vaccines
>
> Stings, bites
>
> Contact allergies (i.e. latex)

> **Box 7.3** Management of acute urticaria
>
> - Remove offending medications or food
> - Treat infectious diseases
> - Start a scheduled nonsedating antihistamine
> - Instruct patient on dose-escalation of nonsedating antihistamines
> - Start an as needed sedating antihistamine
> - Consider use of systemic steroids such as oral prednisone 40–60 mg daily for 5 days or equivalent (pediatrics 1 mg/kg per day times 5 days)

---

determining the cause of urticaria. The most common causes of acute urticaria are outlined in Box 7.2. A careful search for these or other inciting factors should be performed. In most cases of urticaria, no routine laboratory tests are indicated.

Pitfall | **Failure to provide adequate duration of antihistamine and steroid therapy**

The stepwise management of acute urticaria is outlined in Box 7.3. Any identifiable underlying cause should be removed, and infections should be treated, if possible. First-line therapy for urticaria is antihistamines (Table 7.1). Newer H_1 antihistamines are very effective, with minimal side effects. Increasing the dosage of nonsedating H_1 antihistamines up to four-fold is recommended in chronic urticaria; these off-label dosages have improved symptoms from urticaria without increasing

Table 7.1 Oral antihistamines for urticaria. (Data from [28])

Generic name	Adult dosage	Pediatric dosage
Non-sedating antihistamines		
Loratadine	10 mg	2–5 years: 5 mg daily 6–11 years: 10 mg daily
Desloratadine	5 mg daily	6–11 months: 1 mg daily 1–5 years: 1.25 mg daily 6–11 years: 2.5 mg daily
Cetirizine	10 mg daily	6–11 months: 2.5 mg daily 12–23 months: 2.5 mg BID 2–5 years: 2.5–5 mg daily 6–11 years: 5–10 mg daily
Levocetirizine	5 mg daily	6–11 years: 5 mg daily
Fexofenadine	180 mg daily	6–23 months: 15 mg BID 2–11 years: 30 mg BID
Sedating antihistamines		
Diphenhydramine	25–50 mg every 4 h Max: 300 mg/day	2–6 years: 6.25–12.5 mg every 4 h Max: 75 mg/day 6–12 years: 12–25 mg every 4 h Max: 150 mg/day
Cyproheptadine	4 mg TID	2–6 years: 2 mg BID-TID 7–14 years: 4 mg BID-TID
Hydroxyzine	25–50 mg TID-QID	<6 years: 50 mg/day in divided doses >6 years: 50–100 mg/day in divided doses

somnolence [16, 17]. Similar dosing regimens could be used in acute urticaria, though efficacy has not been specifically studied. Newer H_1 antihistamines may be combined with first-generation antihistamines. Patients need to be instructed to take antihistamines on a scheduled basis for 1 to 2 weeks. If a patient fails scheduled antihistamines, adding systemic corticosteroids to a scheduled antihistamine regimen results in decreased itching and more rapid resolution of symptoms. It does not necessarily change the duration of acute urticaria [18].

Pitfall | Failure to treat moderate to severe *Toxicodendron* dermatitis with adequate dose and duration of corticosteroids

The *Toxicodendron* genus of plants includes poison ivy, poison oak, and poison sumac. These plants are the most common cause of allergic contact dermatitis in North America. Up to 50 million Americans are affected each year [19]. Most adults in the United States are clinically *Toxicodendron*-sensitive [19]. Urushiol is a colorless to slightly yellow resin found in all parts of the *Toxicodendron* plant, including the roots, stems, leaves, and fruit. Within minutes of exposure to skin, urushiol begins to penetrate the outer skin layers and bind with cell membranes, initiating a delayed-hypersensitivity dermatitis. Symptoms of itching and erythema begin 24–48 hours after exposure (range 5 hours to 15 days). This is followed by the development of vesicles, bullae, and edema. The severity and distribution of disease depends on the degree of individual sensitization, skin thickness, volume of urushiol, method of contact (direct, burning), and body surface area exposed.

The diagnosis of *Toxicodendron* dermatitis is made by clinical history and examination. Most patients will recall a history of exposure in the last several days. The dermatitis caused by *Toxicodendron* plants is universally pruritic. If the patient is not complaining of itching, other diagnoses must be entertained. On examination, the eruption is asymmetric and exhibits areas of linearity where a plant or fomite rubbed the resin against the skin. Since thinner skin is more sensitive than thicker skin, many patients have involvement on the face, neck, and dorsal extremities with some sparing of palms and soles. In addition, it is important for the acute care provider to recognize that some patients will exhibit a phenomenon known as autoeczematization or id reaction. This occurs when patients have the eruption on areas of the skin both directly exposed to *and* not directly exposed to the plants. The assessment of patients with potential *Toxicodendron* dermatitis should include vital signs and visual inspection to assess the patient for possible secondary bacterial infection or other allergic reaction.

> KEY FACT | On examination, the eruption is asymmetric and exhibits areas of linearity where a plant or fomite rubbed the resin against the skin.

Left untreated, *Toxicodendron* dermatitis can last 3 to 6 weeks. With treatment, symptoms may persist for 2 weeks. The goal of treatment is to reduce the erythema, pruritus, and blistering for the patient. Mild localized disease (e.g. on forearm) may be treated with potent topical corticosteroids for 2 to 3 weeks. The mainstay of therapy is systemic corticosteroids for all but the mildest cases. For adults, prednisone (or equivalent) at a dose of 1–2 mg/kg/day (peds 0.5 mg/kg/day) as a single morning dose for 7–10 days followed by an additional 7–10-day taper is most effective. Intramuscular steroids are also effective but there is some variability in release from the depot. Steroid dose packs do not have sufficient dose or duration and should not be used. If the patient is not treated with a high enough or long enough dose, a steroid-resistant rebound rash may occur. This is clinically similar to a *Toxicodendron* dermatitis but does not respond well to steroid treatment.

> KEY FACT | **Left untreated, Toxicodendron dermatitis can last 3 to 6 weeks. With treatment, symptoms may persist for 2 weeks.**

In addition, simple steps will help ease the skin symptoms. These include: (1) compresses to the skin with cool, damp white cotton towels or long underwear; (2) baths with cornstarch or colloidal oatmeal (put oatmeal in a sock and tie it to avoid clogging pipes); and (3) calamine lotion. For patients with secondary bacterial infection, use oral antibiotics and antiseptic wet dressings. Topical antihistamines, topical antibiotics, and topical anesthetics should be avoided. Oral antihistamines are not particularly helpful for pruritus relief but can be used for their sedative effect.

Common infectious rashes

Pitfall | **Failure to identify and treat early localized Lyme disease to prevent disseminated Lyme**

Lyme disease is a tick-borne illness resulting from the transmission of *Borrelia burgdorferi* to human hosts from the *Ixodes* species of tick, most commonly the deer tick [20]. Most cases are diagnosed in spring and early summer, when ticks are most abundant. Early localized Lyme disease (Stage I) occurs 7 to 10 days after the tick bite and is characterized by flu-like symptoms, headaches, and arthralgias, along with the characteristic *erythema migrans* rash at the site of the tick bite. 75 percent of patients will develop *erythema migrans* which is described as either a macular rash with central clearing or a central red patch, surrounded by normal skin, which is then surrounded by a migrating, erythematous band [20, 21]. Early disseminated disease (Stage II), occurring weeks after exposure, manifests with neurologic and cardiovascular pathology, including meningitis, Bell's palsy, mononeuropathies, myocarditis, and atrioventricular nodal block. Late chronic disease (Stage III) manifests with profound fatigue, polyneuropathy, arthralgias, encephalopathy, and leukoencephalitis [22].

Table 7.2 Treatment of uncomplicated zoster. (Data from [29, 30])

Agent	Name and dosing	Comments
Antivirals*	Acyclovir: 800 mg PO 5×daily×7 days Valacyclovir: 1 gm PO TID×7 days Famciclovir: 500 mg PO TID×7 days	– All therapeutically equivalent, but valacyclovir and famciclovir preferred due to ease of dosing
Steroids**	Prednisone: 60 mg PO daily	– Taper over 2 weeks

*Start within 72 hours of onset of rash

**Avoid in patients with diabetes, hypertension, osteoporosis, and immunodeficiency (ID-1–48)

The acute care provider should know the regional prevalence of Lyme and ascertain a history of potential tick exposure. For patients in an endemic area presenting with symptoms of Lyme and a classic *erythema migrans* rash, no serologic testing is necessary. Treatment can be initiated with 3 weeks of doxycycline 100 mg twice daily or, alternatively, amoxicillin 500 mg three times daily [21]. Patients with symptoms of Lyme but lacking objective findings on evaluation should be referred for serologic testing. Serologic testing is wrought with complexities beyond the scope of this chapter. Importantly, patients reporting tick exposure alone who are asymptomatic and without *erythema migrans*, do not require prophylactic treatment but instead should be monitored for development of symptoms over the next 30 days [22]. If a tick has been attached for less than 24–48 hours, the likelihood of disease transmission is very low [5].

Pitfall | **Failure to identify high-risk patients with zoster who require immediate referral**

Varicella zoster virus (VZV) is a herpes virus causing two distinct syndromes: varicella (chicken pox) and zoster (shingles). Over one million cases of shingles are diagnosed annually in the United States with 30% of individuals developing shingles in their lifetime [23]. After primary infection with chicken pox, VZV becomes latent in the dorsal ganglia root. VZV reactivates when immunity wanes, resulting in the clinical syndrome of shingles [24]. Individuals at risk of developing shingles include those with cancer, organ transplant, human immunodeficiency virus,

or those taking immunosuppressive agents [25]. Advanced age is the most significant risk factor. Two-thirds of patients who get shingles are over 60 years of age, with patients over 75 having the greatest risk [23, 26]. Clinically, shingles begins with a syndrome of malaise, photophobia, and headache followed by dermatomal paresthesias or pain, all of which can precede the rash by as many as 5 days. A dermatomal erythematous maculopapular rash is quickly followed by the development of clustered vesicles which form over a 3- to 5-day period and then crust over. Pain occurs in 95% of patients over 50, and it is often severe [27]. Post-herpetic neuralgia, defined as persistent pain beyond 120 days, is one of the most debilitating complications of shingles [26].

Diagnosis of shingles can usually be made clinically by the history and the distinctive rash. Confirmatory VZV polymerase chain reaction testing can be performed and is the most sensitive technique currently available. Treatment of uncomplicated zoster is outlined in Table 7.2.

High-risk patients with zoster requiring immediate referral and transfer would include those with fever, secondary cellulitis, immunosuppression, affected by multiple dermatomes, or potential involvement of the eye (first division of the trigeminal nerve).

Pitfall | **Failure to prescribe adequate and appropriate topical corticosteroids**

Many skin problems seen in the acute care setting can be adequately treated with topical corticosteroids. These include atopic dermatitis, seborrheic dermatitis, nummular eczema, psoriasis, and local-

Table 7.3 Topical corticosteroids.

Generic name	Vehicle: Strength
Low potency	
Desonide	Cream: 0.05%
	Lotion: 0.05%
	Ointment: 0.05%
Hydrocortisone	Cream: 0.5%, 1%, 2.5%
	Lotion: 1%, 2.5%
	Ointment: 0.5%, 1%, 2.5%
Medium potency	
Fluocinolone acetonide	Cream: 0.01%, 0.025%
	Ointment: 0.025%
	Solution: 0.01%
Triamcinolone acetonide	Cream: 0.025%, 0.1%, 0.5%
	Lotion: 0.025%, 0.1%
	Ointment: 0.025%, 0.05%, 0.1%, 0.5%
High potency	
Desoximetasone	Cream: 0.05%, 0.25%
	Gel: 0.05%
	Ointment: 0.25%
Fluocinonide	Cream: 0.05%
	Emollient cream: 0.05%
	Gel: 0.05%
	Ointment: 0.05%
	Solution: 0.05%

Data from MICROMEDIX Healthcare Series [28].

Table 7.4 Estimating the necessary amount of topical corticosteroid for adults.

Area	Amount for twice daily application for 2 weeks
Face and neck	36 g
Trunk (front and back)	186 g
One arm	48 g
One hand	17 g
One leg	81 g
One foot	25 g

Data from Long and Finlay [31].

ized contact dermatitis. When selecting a topical corticosteroid for use, several factors must be considered. (1) What potency should be used? (2) What vehicle should be used? (3) What quantity should be dispensed? There are several classification systems that rank topical corticosteroids by potency. In general, low potency corticosteroids may be used on all body areas on children and on thin or occluded areas on adults (face, intertriginous, genitals). Medium potency steroids are ideal for the trunk and extremities of teens and adults. High potency steroids should be reserved for thick-skinned areas (palms, soles), lichenified areas, and for diseases that are more corticosteroid resistant. Because of the vast number of products available, it is reasonable for the clinician to familiarize themselves with one or two from each category for use (Table 7.3).

Second, vehicle choice is an important consideration. The most common vehicles include ointments, creams, and solutions. Ointments are water-in-oil emulsions, making them soothing, occlusive, and most effective. While greasy, they are least irritating of all vehicles and will not sting when applied to inflamed skin. Creams are oil-in-water preparations that have alcohol and often propylene glycol in them. Because of this, they are not as greasy but can be irritating to cracked or fissured skin. They work well for acute and weeping dermatoses. Solutions have high amounts of alcohol, making them reasonable choices for the scalp and densely hairy areas.

Finally, it is important to consider how much body surface area is involved as this will dictate the quantity of topical corticosteroid a patient will require for therapy. Providers routinely fail to prescribe adequate amounts of topical steroids. Table 7.4 depicts the amounts required for twice daily application for 2 weeks.

The most common negative side effect of short-term (2 weeks) topical corticosteroid use is mild, local skin irritation. Other side effects such as skin atrophy and clinically significant hypothalamic pituitary axis suppression are unlikely with short-term use.

Summary

The acute care provider must employ a rational approach to efficiently, safely, and effectively manage the patient who presents with a rash in the acute care setting. A series of three questions, outlined in detail in Figure 7.1, can help to define this approach. Using these questions, providers can avoid pitfalls in the management of rashes.

Pearls to improve patient outcome

• Initiate treatment and transport immediately to a referral center of patients who present with clinical toxicity, fever, vital sign abnormalities, petechial rashes, or rashes with extensive mucosal involvement, skin sloughing or blistering.

• Always examine carefully for mucosal membrane involvement; significant conjunctival, oral, or genital involvement should alert the provider of possible SJS or TEN.

• Aggressively incise and drain CA-MRSA abscesses, as infection is likely to persist if antibiotic therapy is used alone.

• Secure a definitive airway early in patients with angioedema of the upper airway.

• Instruct all patients with acute urticaria to take a scheduled nonsedating antihistamine.

• Prescribe 14–21 days of systemic corticosteroids for moderate to severe *Toxicodendron* dermatitis.

• Prescribe a large enough quantity of topical corticosteroids to cover the affected body surface area for 2 weeks.

References

1 Freiman A, Borsuk D, Sasseville D. Dermatologic emergencies. *CMAJ* 2005; **173**(11): 1317–1319.

2 Centers for Disease Control and Prevention. Tickborne rickettsial diseases: Rocky Mountain spotted fever. http://www.cdc.gov/ticks/diseases/rocky_mountain_spotted_fever/. Accesses January 21, 2011.

3 Wolff K, Johnson RA, Fitzpatrick TB. *Fitzpatrick's Color Atlas and Synopsis of Clinical Dermatology* (5th edn.). McGraw-Hill: New York, NY, 2005: pp. 756–758.

4 O'Reilly M, Paddock C, Elchos B, *et al.* Physician knowledge of the diagnosis and management of Rocky Mountain spotted fever: Mississippi, 2002. *Ann NY Acad Sci* 2003; **990**: 295–301.

5 Browne BJ, Edwards B, Rogers RL. Dermatologic emergencies. *Prim Care Clin Office Pract* 2006; **33**: 685–695.

6 Ferguson LE, Hormann MD, Parks DK, *et al.* Neisseria meningitidis: presentation, treatment, and prevention. *J Pediatr Health Care* 2002; **16**(3): 119–124.

7 Salzman MB, Rubin LG. Meningococcemia. *Infect Dis Clin North Am* 1996; **10**(4): 709–725.

8 Parrillo SJ. Stevens–Johnson syndrome and toxic epidermal necrolysis. *Curr Allergy Asthma Rep* 2007; **7**(4): 243–247.

9 Usatine RP, Sandy N. Dermatologic emergencies. *Am Fam Phys* 2010; **82**(7): 773–780.

10 Gannon T. Dermatologic emergencies. When early recognition can be lifesaving. *Postgrad Med* 1994; **96**(1): 67–70, 73–75, 79.

11 Ahrenholz DH. Necrotizing soft-tissue infections. *Surg Clin North Am* 1988; **68**(1): 199–214.

12 Simonart T, Simonart JM, Derdelinckx I, *et al.* Value of standard laboratory tests for the early recognition of group A beta-hemolytic streptococcal necrotizing fasciitis. *Clin Infect Dis* 2001; **32**(1): E9–E12.

13 Centers for Disease Control and Prevention. Group A streptococcal (GAS) disease. http://www.cdc.gov/ncidod/dbmd/diseaseinfo/groupastreptococcal_t.htm. Accessed January 21, 2011.

14 Frigas E, Park MA. Acute urticaria and angioedema: diagnostic and treatment considerations. *Am J Clin Dermatol* 2009; **10**(4): 239–250.

15 Zuberbier T, Blindslev-Jensen C, Canonica W, *et al.* EAACI/GA2LEN/EDF guideline: definition, classification and diagnosis of urticaria. *Allergy* 2006; **61**(3): 316–320.

16 Hindmarch I, Shamsi Z, Kimber S: An evaluation of the effects of high-dose fexofenadine on the central nervous system: a double-blind, placebo-controlled study in healthy volunteers. *Clin Exp Allergy* 2002; **32**(1): 133–139.

17 Staevska M, Popov TA, Kralimarkova T, *et al.* The effectiveness of Levocetirizine and desloratadine in up to 4 times conventional doses in difficult-to-treat urticaria. *J Allergy Clin Immunol* 2010; **125**(3): 676–682.

18 Poon M, Reid C. Best evidence topics reports. Oral corticosteroids in acute urticaria. *Emerg Med J* 2004; **21**(1): 76–77.

19 Gladman AC. Toxicodendron dermatitis: Poison Ivy, Oak, and Sumac. *Wilderness Environ Med* 2006; **17**(2): 120–128.

20 McGinley-Smith DE, Tsao SS. Dermatoses from ticks. *J Am Acad Dermatol* 2003; **49**(3): 363–392 [quiz 393–396].

21 Bratton RL, Corey R. Tick-borne disease. *Am Fam Phys* 2005; **71**(12): 2323–2330.

22 DePietropaolo DL, Powers JH, Gill JM *et al.* Diagnosis of Lyme disease. *Am Fam Phys* 2005; **72**(2): 297–304.

23 Harpaz R, Ortega-Sanchez IR, Seward JF. Prevention of herpes zoster: recommendations of the Advisory Committee of Immunization Practices (ACIP). *MMWR* 2008; **57**(RR-5): 1–30.

24 Gnann JW Jr., Whitley RJ. Herpes zoster. *N Engl J Med* 2002; **347**(5): 340–346.

25 Straus SE, Reinhold W, Smith HA, *et al.* Endonuclease analysis of viral DNA from varicella and subsequent zoster infections in the same patient. *N Engl J Med* 1984; **311**(21): 1362–4.

26 Whitley RJ: A 70-year-old woman with shingles. Review of herpes zoster. *JAMA* 2009; **302**(1): 73–80.

27 Gilden DH, Kleinschmidt-DeMasters BK, LaGuardia JJ, *et al.* Neurologic complications of the reactivation of varicella-zoster virus. *N Engl J Med* 2000; **342**(9): 635–645.

28 MICROMEDIX Healthcare Series. http://www.thomsonhc.com/hcs/librarian. Accessed on January 20, 2011.

29 Tyring SK, Beutner KR, Tucker BA, *et al.* Antiviral therapy for herpes zoster: randomized, controlled clinical trial of valacyclovir and famciclovir therapy in immunocompetent patients 50 years and older. *Arch Fam Med* 2000; **9**(9): 863–869.

30 Wood MJ, Johnson RW, McKendrick MW, *et al.* A randomized trial of acyclovir for 7 days or 21 days with and without prednisolone for treatment of acute herpes zoster. *N Engl J Med* 1994; **330**(13): 896–900.

31 Long CC, Finlay AY. The finger-tip unit – a new practical measure. *Clin Exp Dermatol* 1991; **16**(6): 444–447.

CHAPTER 8

Management of Common Infections

Siamak Moayedi and Mercedes Torres
Department of Emergency Medicine, University of Maryland School of Medicine, Baltimore, MD, USA

Introduction

The management of common infectious diseases is central to the practice of urgent care medicine. Acute care providers are challenged to identify the varying manifestations of some of these infectious diseases and treat them accordingly. In all cases, providers are faced with the task of choosing appropriate antibiotics when indicated, while withholding antibiotics in instances where they are not needed. The goal of this chapter is to review some of the most common infectious diagnoses in urgent care settings with a focus on their accurate diagnoses and appropriate treatments.

Pitfall | **Inappropriate treatment of skin and soft tissue infections (SSTIs) in the age of community-acquired methicillin-resistant *Staphylococcus aureus* (CA-MRSA)**

Recent epidemiologic data demonstrates that greater than 50% of SSTIs at major medical centers in the US were a result of CA-MRSA [1]. Patients can present with furuncles, folliculitis, impetigo, purulent cellulitis, carbuncles, paronychia, abscesses, and necrotizing fasciitis. The role of CA-MRSA in nonpurulent cellulitis is less clear [2]. Given the increasing frequency of CA-MRSA infections, the Infectious Disease Society of America (IDSA) has released guidelines for acute care providers which offer recommendations for evidence-based management of SSTIs. The key points of these guidelines are summarized in Table 8.1.

Several randomized controlled trials have demonstrated the utility of incision and drainage (I&D) alone in treating simple cutaneous abscesses [1, 3]. A recent study compared the use of trimethoprim-sulfamethoxazole (TMP-SMX) and placebo in adults for 7 days subsequent to I&D of simple cutaneous abscesses, and found no difference in the rate of treatment failure. The literature on the utility of antibiotics post-I&D in pediatric patients demonstrates similar results. In nontoxic appearing, afebrile children aged 3 months to 18 years, treatment failure rates with TMP-SMX versus placebo after I&D were comparable at 4–5% [3]. Therefore, the current recommendation for the management of simple abscesses in uncomplicated patients is I&D only [4].

> KEY FACT | **Incision and drainage alone is effective for treatment of simple cutaneous CA-MRSA abscesses in uncomplicated patients.**

Complicated SSTIs are characterized by more severe disease, systemic symptoms, and progressive examination findings. Any abscess in an immunocompromised patient or located in an area not amenable to I&D should be considered complicated as well. Antimicrobial therapy is indicated in these cases (see Table 8.1) and appropriate antibiotic choice is of utmost importance. SSTIs presenting as classic CA-MRSA infections, such as simple abscesses, furuncles or carbuncles, should be

Urgent Care Emergencies: Avoiding the Pitfalls and Improving the Outcomes, First Edition.
Edited by Deepi G. Goyal and Amal Mattu.
© 2012 John Wiley & Sons, Ltd. Published 2012 by John Wiley & Sons, Ltd.

Table 8.1 Recommended initial treatment of SSTIs based on patient and infection characteristics

Recommended initial treatment	SSTI and patient characteristics
I&D ONLY	Simple abscess in otherwise healthy patient
I&D+antibiotics for CA-MRSA	Abscess with one or more of the following:
	• Severe or extensive disease
	• Progressive associated cellulitis
	• Signs of systemic illness
	• High risk comorbidities or immunosuppression
	• Extremes of age
	• Problematic location for I&D (hands, face, genitals)
	• Associated septic phlebitis
	• Ineffective previous I&D
Empiric antibiotics for CA-MRSA without I&D	Cellulitis with one or more of the following:
	• Purulence but no abscess amenable to drainage
	• No purulence but no response to beta-lactam treatment
	• Signs of systemic illness
Empiric antibiotics for beta-hemolytic strep	Nonpurulent cellulitis

Data from Liu *et al.* [4]

Table 8.2 IDSA oral antibiotic recommendations for coverage of SSTIs in outpatients

Likely organism	Agents recommended
CA-MRSA	• Trimethoprim-sulfamethoxazole (TMP-SMX)
	• Clindamycin
	• Doxycycline or minocycline
	• Linezolid
CA-MRSA+Beta-Hemolytic Strep	• TMP-SMX+beta-lactam*
	• Clindamycin
	• Doxycycline or minocycline+beta-lactam*
	• Linezolid

*Beta-lactam agents include penicillins, cephalosporins and carbapenems.
Data from Liu *et al.* [4]

Table 8.3 Antimicrobial agents and dosing for outpatient management of CA-MRSA SSTIs

Antimicrobial	Dosing
Trimethoprim-sulfamethoxazole (TMP-SMX)	1–2 tabs PO BID
Clindamycin	150 mg–450 mg PO q6 h
Doxycycline	100 mg PO BID
Minocycline	100 mg PO BID (first dose 200 mg)
Rifampin	300 mg PO BID (cannot be used as monotherapy)
Linezolid	400 mg PO q12 h

Data from Liu *et al.* [4]

treated with an agent that covers CA-MRSA with appropriate dosing (see Tables 8.2 and 8.3 for specific antibiotics and dosing). Notably, while rifampin is very effective against MRSA, it must be combined with TMP-SMX, doxycycline, or minocycline to ensure that rapid resistance does not develop. Furthermore, rifampin causes the unpleasant side effect of discoloration of body fluids and decreases the effectiveness of oral contraception medications [5]. Another complicating factor is the increasing prevalence of inducible resistance to clindamycin, which is indicated on culture results as resistance to erythromycin. These issues should be considered prior to prescribing antibiotics [5].

No prospective human trials exist to support the recommendation of increased TMP-SMX dosing to two tablets orally twice daily, however the theory supporting this practice focuses on increasing serum levels to an effective concentration in the area of the abscess. The risks of this increased dosing include more frequent side effects or adverse reactions [5].

SSTIs which could also involve beta-hemolytic streptococcal infection, most notably purulent cellulitis or extensive cellulitis surrounding an abscessed or necrotizing area, require appropriate coverage for both CA-MRSA and strep, as indicated in Table 8.2. Nonpurulent cellulitis alone is not commonly associated with CA-MRSA, therefore antibiotics covering strep alone are recommended. While clindamycin is able to provide strep and CA-MRSA coverage, TMP-SMX, doxycycline and minocycline all require the addition of a beta-lactam (e.g. amoxicillin or cephalexin) to the regimen for strep coverage [4].

Decolonization of patients has been proposed in an attempt to address the increasing frequency and recurrence of CA-MRSA SSTIs. CA-MRSA most frequently colonizes the nares, although the respiratory tract, perineum, groin, axilla, and urinary tract have all been implicated. Risk factors for CA-MRSA colonization include previous hospitalization, age greater than 65, indwelling catheters, a history of diabetes, antibiotic use, hemodialysis and close contact with a colonized person. The two indications for MRSA decolonization are attempted eradication of the organism in patients with multiple previous infections, and attempted control of MRSA transmission among a closely associated, well-defined cohort of patients, for example household contacts [6].

> KEY FACT | **MRSA decolonization of patients can be effective in the short term, but does not decrease MRSA currences in the long term.**

The only agent that has shown any efficacy in MRSA decolonization is 2% mupirocin ointment. Recent studies demonstrate that mupirocin ointment is effective in short-term decolonization efforts. However, the overall reinfection rates were similar 2 months subsequent to attempted decolonization [7]. It has been recommended for use intranasally twice daily for 5 to 10 days in select patient populations described in the previous paragraph [4, 6].

> **Box 8.1** Areas for focus of patient education to prevent recurrent CA-MRSA infections
>
> - *Keep draining wounds covered* with clean, dry bandages
> - *Maintain good personal hygiene* including regular bathing and hand washing with soap and water or an alcohol-based hand gel, especially after contact with wound
> - *Avoid reusing or sharing personal items* (i.e. razors, towels) that have contacted infected skin
> - *Focus cleaning efforts on high-touch areas* that may contact bare skin or uncovered infections (i.e. door knobs, phones, counter tops, toilet seats)
>
> Data from Liu *et al.* [4]

Chlorhexadine body washes for 5–14 days have shown possible efficacy only in conjunction with mupirocin [4, 6]. Other topical methods and all oral regimens have not proven effective and are generally not recommended [4, 6].

Efforts aimed at preventing the recurrence of CA-MRSA infections have focused on patient education. The important points are summarized in Box 8.1 [4].

Pitfall | **Misdiagnosis of an aggressive soft tissue infection as cellulitis**

Uncomplicated cellulitis in a patient without immunosupression is commonly treated with outpatient antibiotics. It is imperative to always consider more aggressive soft tissue infections as delay in diagnosis and management of necrotizing soft tissue infections (NSTI) will lead to significant morbidity and mortality. NSTIs lead to rapidly progressive tissue destruction and have a mortality of greater than 20% [8]. The difficulty in diagnosis of this entity is related to the pathogens' ability to rapidly and widely spread along tissue planes without significant involvement of the skin surface. The most common pathogens leading to NSTIs are group A streptococcus, *Staphylococcus aureus*, *Clostridium perfringes*, and various mixtures of anaerobic organisms. The subtypes of these bacteria capable of producing necrotizing fasciitis possess exotoxins which cause tissue destruction.

KEY FACT | **Necrotizing fasciitis rapidly spreads along tissue planes without significant skin surface involvement.**

Distinguishing an early NSTI which would require emergent surgical debridement and aggressive parenteral antibiotics from an uncomplicated cellulitis is challenging. Clinical signs that are specific for NSTI include the presence of bullae, ecchymosis, crepitus, and superficial anesthesia of the skin. Unfortunately, these signs occur in the minority of cases and develop late in the process of the disease. Clinical clues that can help to differentiate between an NSTI and cellulitis early in the process include pain out of proportion to the extent of skin involvement; edema extending past the skin erythema; and a history of immunosuppression. Patients with signs concerning for a NSTI should be referred immediately to an emergency department to initiate emergent care and diagnostic measures.

Pitfall | Misdiagnosis of deep venous thrombosis as cellulitis

Cellulitis in the lower leg is characterized by signs and symptoms that may be similar to those of a deep vein thrombosis (DVT), such as warmth, pain, and swelling. Given the significant mortality associated with untreated DVT it is important to make an accurate diagnosis. Although fever and chills are more common with cellulitis, these findings can occur with DVT. Lymphangitis and tender adenopathy in the ipsilateral groin support the diagnosis of cellulitis. Furthermore, cellulitis will have sharply demarcated and advancing erythematous borders.

In one study of ED patients presenting with lower extremity pain and swelling with an initial impression of DVT versus cellulitis, 66% were diagnosed with cellulitis, 17.5% had a confirmed DVT, 2% were diagnosed with both cellulitis and DVT, and 16.5% were diagnosed with another entity such as Baker's cyst or superficial thrombosis. Patients with a diagnosis of cellulitis were more likely to have a history of diabetes. Interestingly, patients with leukocytosis were less likely to have cellulitis. This affirms the futility of ordering CBCs

in an attempt to differentiate between cellulitis and DVT [9]. Studies documenting the prevalence of both cellulitis and acute DVT in the same lower extremity range from 0–15% [10]. It is plausible that the edema caused by an occlusive DVT can place patients at risk for developing cellulitis. In this scenario, a careful history will likely illustrate the presence of edema prior to the secondary infection.

KEY FACT | **The prevalence of both cellulitis and acute DVT in the same extremity is 0–15%.**

Pitfall | Overuse of antibiotics for upper respiratory infections

The majority of antibiotics prescribed in acute care practice are for upper respiratory infections (colds), sinusitis, pharyngitis and bronchitis. For most of these conditions, antibiotics do not provide any benefit, while contributing to antibiotic resistance and placing the patient at risk of medication side effects. Furthermore, the prescription rates for expensive and broad spectrum antibiotics have been increasing, creating an undue financial burden on patients and healthcare systems.

There is ample evidence-based literature guiding the appropriate management of these common maladies (listed below). However, the trend for antibiotic misuse continues due to a variety of pressures including patients who insist on antibiotics (reinforced from previous prescriptions), lack of time to explain why antibiotics are unnecessary, commercial advertising from drug companies and providers who are overly cautious [11]. There are a variety of ways to decrease inappropriate antibiotic prescription. Using several methods in combination works better than using one method alone [11]. The U.S. Centers for Disease Control (CDC) campaign "Get smart: know when antibiotics work" (www. cdc.gov/getsmart) provides a wealth of information from treatment guidelines to patient information brochures regarding the futility of antibiotics for the treatment of the aforementioned common complaints. A key concept in the recommendations is that patient satisfaction with their care for these conditions is predominantly based on provider–patient communication, rather than antibiotic prescription.

Box 8.2 Communication strategies to decrease antibiotic prescription

- *Provide a specific diagnosis* to help patients feel validated. For example, say "viral bronchitis" instead of referring to an illness as "just a virus."
- *Recommend symptomatic relief.* Often, patients request an antibiotic because they think it will help them feel better without realizing that effective symptomatic therapies can provide the relief they are seeking.
- *Share normal findings* as you go through your exam. For example, let patients know that their lungs sound clear. This reassures the patient that the illness may not be as severe as they thought and may make them more open to the idea that they do not need an antibiotic.
- *Discuss potential side effects* of antibiotic use, including adverse events and resistance.
- *Explain to the patient what to expect* over the next few days. This can help them feel reassured and empowered. Give patients a plan of action in case symptoms do change or become worse.

Data from Centers for Disease Control and Prevention, www.cdc.gov/getsmart

> KEY FACT | **Patient satisfaction is predominantly based on provider–patient communication rather than antibiotic prescription.**

Five communication strategies endorsed by the CDC are listed in Box 8.2. It is often helpful to personalize the risk of antibiotic use by highlighting common side effects such as gastrointestinal upset, yeast infection or the development of resistant strains of pathogens risking treatment failures for future serious bacterial infections. Other strategies include giving patients printed material supporting your decision not to prescribe antibiotics. Finally, delaying a prescription by asking the patient not to fill it for a set number of days is a viable method of decreasing antibiotic use.

Principles for appropriate antibiotic therapy for evaluation and treatment of bronchitis, pharyngitis, sinusitis, and upper respiratory infections are summarized in the following section. These guidelines apply to otherwise healthy adults and exclude the elderly and patients with comorbid conditions such as immunosuppression or emphysema.

Bronchitis

The evaluation of adults with an acute cough illness should focus on ruling out pneumonia. In the healthy, non-elderly adult, pneumonia is uncommon in the absence of vital sign abnormalities or asymmetrical lung sounds, therefore chest radiography is usually not indicated. In patients with cough lasting 3 weeks or longer, chest radiography is warranted in the absence of other known causes. Routine antibiotic treatment of uncomplicated bronchitis is not recommended, regardless of the duration of the cough [12].

Pharyngitis

Group A beta hemolytic streptococcus (GABHS) is the etiologic agent in approximately 10% of adult cases of pharyngitis. The large majority of adults with acute pharyngitis (including GABHS) have a self-limiting illness. The benefits of antibiotic treatment of adult pharyngitis are limited to those patients with GABHS infection. All patients with pharyngitis should be offered appropriate doses of analgesics, antipyretics and other supportive care. Clinically screen all adult patients with pharyngitis for the presence of the four Centor criteria [13]: (1) fever or recent history of fever; (2) tonsillar exudates; (3) absence of cough; and (4) tender anterior cervical lymphadenopathy. Test patients with two or three criteria using a rapid antigen test. Limit antibiotic therapy to patients with a positive test or patients with four criteria. If a rapid antigen test is unavailable, limit antibiotic therapy to patients with three or four criteria. The preferred antibiotic for treatment of acute GABHS pharyngitis is penicillin [14]. Corticosteroids are not indicated in the routine treatment of exudative pharyngitis and only provide a small reduction in the time to pain relief in GABHS pharyngitis [15].

> KEY FACT | **Corticosteroids are only beneficial for exudative pharyngitis caused by group A beta hemolytic streptococcus.**

Sinusitis

ost cases of acute sinusitis are due to uncomplicated viral infections. The clinical diagnosis of acute bacterial sinusitis should be reserved for patients with sinusitis symptoms lasting 7 days or more and who have maxillary facial/tooth pain or tenderness (especially when unilateral) and purulent nasal secretions. Patients who have sinusitis symptoms for less than 7 days are unlikely to have a bacterial infection. Initial treatment should be with the most narrow-spectrum agent that is active against the likely pathogens, *Streptococcus pneumoniae* and *Haemophilus influenza* [16].

Upper respiratory tract infections

An upper respiratory tract infection is defined as an acute infection that is typically viral in origin, and in which sinus, pharyngeal, and lower airway symptoms, although frequently present, are not prominent. Antibiotic treatment of nonspecific upper respiratory infections in adults does not expedite illness resolution or prevent complications, and is therefore not recommended. Purulent secretions in the nares and throat or change in color from yellow to green neither predicts bacterial infection nor benefits from antibiotic treatment [17].

> KEY FACT | **Change in color of sputum from yellow to green neither predicts bacterial infection nor benefits from antibiotics.**

Pitfall | **Failure to diagnose and appropriately treat (*C. difficile*) in patients presenting with diarrhea**

An increasing number of patients ultimately diagnosed with *Clostridium difficile* infection are presenting without a history of traditional risk factors, such as recent use of antibiotics or hospitalization. Other sources of *C. difficile* thought to possibly be responsible for the emergence of this new strain of community-acquired *C. difficile* (CACD) can include soil, household pets, food, or second hand exposure to other colonized individuals [18]. Increased community colonization rates and exposure to asymptomatic carriers have been identified as other, less direct sources of the spread of CACD [19].

Recent studies have shown that the incidence of CACD in the U.S. ranges from 3.2 to 7.6 cases per 100,000 people per year. In these studies, almost half of the patients with CACD had not received any antibiotics in the preceding one month prior to diagnosis. Overall, when patient characteristics were analyzed, it appears that patients presenting with diarrhea from CACD are younger than the traditional *C. difficile* population and have less severe clinical disease [19]. While patients with a history of prior hospitalizations and antibiotic use (especially clindamycin or a fluoroqinolone) remain at increased risk of *C. difficile*, other risk factors such as the use of proton pump inhibitors (PPIs), a history of concurrent renal failure, and a history of irritable bowel disease (IBD), have been identified in patients with CDAD [18, 19].

> KEY FACT | **32% of patients with CACD have not been exposed to antibiotics in the 90 days prior to symptom development and 25% have no recent predisposing conditions or exposures.**

The changing epidemiology of patients diagnosed with CDAD raises the importance of considering and testing for CDAD in the urgent care setting. Any patient suffering from greater than three watery stools per day for at least 2 days may be diagnosed with CDAD and testing should be considered [18].

When initiating therapy directed at CDAD, metronidazole remains the medication of choice for an initial episode or first recurrence due to its effectiveness and low cost. In addition, metronidazole reduces the risk of patients developing vancomycin resistant enterococcus (VRE) [20]. Recurrences often occur within 1–10 days of the completion of initial antibiotics [21, 20]. When multiple recurrences are involved, resistance to metronidazole can develop, therefore oral vancomycin is recommended. There is no evidence to support the use of probiotics such as Lactobacillus in these cases [18, 20].

Pitfall | **Over-reliance on urine dipstick results in treating women for simple urinary tract infections (UTIs)**

Dysuria and urinary frequency are common urgent care complaints in female patients. The decision regarding treatment of these symptoms with antibiotics can be difficult, as acute care providers must weigh the risks of inappropriate antibiotic treatment against patient expectations. A urine dipstick can be helpful in diagnosing UTIs in women with positive nitrates or leukocytes, but there are many patients with typical symptoms and nondiagnostic dipstick results.

> KEY FACT | **Empiric antibiotics for dysuria and urinary frequency can decrease the duration of symptoms irrespective of urine dipstick results.**

One recent prospective double-blinded randomized placebo-controlled clinical trial assessed the value of antibiotics for women between 16 and 50 presenting with symptoms of dysuria and frequency, but negative urine dipsticks results. Women in this trial were assigned to receive 3 days of trimethoprim or placebo. The women treated with trimethoprim had 2 fewer days of dysuria and 4 fewer days of constitutional symptoms such as fever and chills.

These results demonstrate that empiric antibiotics for dysuria and urinary frequency are justified to decrease the duration of symptoms in cases of suspected uncomplicated UTI irrespective of the urine dipstick results. Clearly, this information should be weighed against the risks of adverse medication reactions, super-infection, and bacterial resistance to antibiotics in a given community [22].

Pitfall | Confusion of scabies infestation with bed bug infestation

Bed bugs (*Cimex lectularius*) are wingless, red-brown, blood-sucking insects that grow up to 7 mm in length with a lifespan of between 4 months and 1 year. They typically hide during daylight and emerge nocturnally to feed. They are capable of anesthetizing the skin which allows them to take a blood meal without detection. Bed bug bites are occasionally observed as linear (groups of three), erythematous and pruritic lesions ranging from macules to wheals resembling mosquito bites [23]. Symptomatic therapy with antihistamines and topical steroids is beneficial. Eradication requires elimination of the bugs from bedding and other hiding places. Powerful insecticides and professional exterminators are often required for this task.

Scabies is caused by microscopic mites too small to be seen without magnification. They burrow into the superficial layer of the dermis and lay eggs. Scabies is spread by direct and prolonged skin-to-skin contact. It occurs most commonly in institutional environments such as homeless shelters, schools, and nursing homes. Patients exposed for the first time do not develop any symptoms for 2–6 weeks after infestation. Infested patients are capable of transmitting the mites during this asymptomatic period. Patients with prior exposure to mite antigens will develop pruritis and skin findings between 1 and 4 days post-infestation.

The intense itching and skin rash is caused by a delayed allergic reaction to the feces and proteins of the mites. Itching is intensified at night time and during physical activity when core temperature is elevated. The rash appears as nonspecific small papules which may be diffuse or limited to areas of the body where two layers of skin rub or touch each other (example: between fingers, armpits, buttocks, etc). Occasionally, tiny burrows can be visualized as raised lines on the skin surface. However burrows may be difficult to find. The most common complication is super-infection of the skin caused by traumatic excoriation. The diagnosis of scabies is clinical as skin evaluation for the mites has a low yield.

Treatment is recommended for all patient contacts with prolonged skin to skin exposures (recall that patients infested for the first time may be asymptomatic for up to 6 weeks). The rash and pruritis may persist for 2 weeks post-treatment. First line therapy is topical 5% permethrin cream applied for 8 hours to the body. Lindane solution is not suggested as a first-line therapy due to its potential for neurotoxicity. The absorption of lindane is enhanced in cases of severe excoriation. Lindane is contraindicated during pregnancy and in children less than 5 years of age. Refractory and severe cases can be simultaneously treated with oral ivermectin [23]. Bedding and clothing used by the patient can be placed in a dryer and exposed to high heat, or bagged for 3 days as mites are unable to survive without skin exposure for that length of time.

KEY FACT | **Scabies mites are unable to survive without skin exposure for more than 3 days.**

The difference between bed bug bites and scabies can be subtle. In general, bed bug bites often occur in a linear pattern. Furthermore, bed bugs do not burrow under the dermis and thus are not contagious unless hiding in clothing or bedding. Scabies mites are not visible to the naked eye, whereas beg bugs can be seen. The pruritis associated with bed bug bites is improved with warm water, whereas it is intensified if related to scabies.

Pitfall | **Indiscriminate use of antibiotics as prophylaxis after tick bites**

Lyme disease, caused by the spirochete *Borrelia burgderferi* is transmitted by the Ixodes tick commonly known as the deer tick. Most cases of Lyme disease in the U.S. occur in the northeast, from Maryland to New England, as well as parts of Minnesota, Wisconsin, and Michigan [24]. Due to aggressive Lyme disease information campaigns, patients often present to acute care facilities with concerns regarding tick exposure ranging from the observation of a tick on the skin, to the complaint that a tick is embedded in their skin. Routine use of antibiotics to prevent Lyme disease is not recommended because of the overall low risk of transmission (1–3%) [24].

KEY FACT | **Transmission of Lyme disease requires tick attachment and engorgement for greater than 36 hours.**

Merely seeing a tick or even having one attached for less than 36 hours is not an indication for treatment. The spirochetes need time to replicate and multiply in the gut of the tick before they can move to its salivary gland in order to be regurgitated into the patient's bloodstream. This process takes more than 36–48 hours and necessitates engorgement of the tick with blood.

Prophylaxis is recommended if the criteria in Box 8.3 are met. If the patient meets criteria for prophylaxis, a single 200-mg dose of doxycycline is effective in preventing Lyme disease [25]. There is no indication for serum testing as antibodies to

Box 8.3 Criteria for Lyme prophylaxis of tick bites

- The tick is identified to be an Ixodes species.
- The exposure was in a Lyme endemic region.
- The tick was attached for more than 36 hours and was engorged.
- The patient has no contraindications to doxycycline therapy (children younger than 8 and pregnant women).

B. burgderferi antigens do not form for several weeks. Ticks that are embedded in the skin must be removed ensuring that there is no compression of the gut. Techniques such as squeezing or burning are discouraged as they may increase the risk of transmission. The correct method for removing a tick involves the use of fine tweezers, grasping the tick as closely as possible to the head and pulling straight out without twisting. If a piece of the head is retained, there is no indication for aggressive measures such as coring the skin. Simply leave the head in place and it will eventually be pushed out by the skin.

Regardless of antibiotic prophylaxis, patients should be instructed to look for the classic erythema migrans rash which occurs in 80% of Lyme infections. The rash can occur any time within the first month of exposure and once present rapidly expands into the typical target appearance. It is possible for the rash to be uniformly erythematous and may be pruritic or painful. The presence of this rash necessitates Lyme disease treatment (doxycycline or amoxicillin for 10–14 days).

Pearls to improve patient outcomes
- Antibiotics for CA-MRSA are not indicated for the management of uncomplicated abscesses after I&D.
- Consider necrotizing fasciitis when there is pain out of proportion to the extent of skin involvement or edema extends past the cellulitis margins.
- Do not rely on a white blood cell count to differentiate between DVT and cellulitis.
- Personalize the risk of antibiotic use by highlighting common side effects and the development of resistance leading to treatment failures in the future.
- Do not prescribe corticosteroids for symptom relief in exudative pharyngitis caused by viruses.

- Patients without a history of recent antibiotic use or hospitalization are still at risk of diarrhea from community-acquired *C. difficile*.
- Symptomatic women with negative urine dipstick results benefit from a short course of antibiotics for UTIs.
- Consider the diagnosis of bed bugs over scabies if the patient reports seeing bugs and the pruritis improves with warm water.
- Deer tick exposures for less than 36 hours do not require Lyme disease prophylaxis.

References

1 Schmitz GR, Bruner D, Pitotti R, *et al.* Randomized controlled trial of trimethoprim-sulfamethoxazole for uncomplicated skin abscesses in patients at risk for community-associated methicillin-resistant Staphylococcus aureus infection. *Ann Emerg Med* 2010; **56**(3): 283–287.

2 Wallin TR, Hern HG, Frazee BW. Community-associated methicillin-resistant Staphylococcus aureus. *Emerg Med Clin North Am* 2008; **26**(2): 431–455, ix.

3 Duong M, Markwell S, Peter J, Barenkamp S. Randomized, controlled trial of antibiotics in the management of community-acquired skin abscesses in the pediatric patient. *Ann Emerg Med* 2010; **55**(5): 401–407.

4 Liu C, Bayer A, Cosgrove SE, *et al.* Clinical Practice Guidelines by the Infectious Diseases Society of America for the Treatment of Methicillin-Resistant *Staphylococcus Aureus* Infections in Adults and Children: Executive Summary. *Clin Infect Dis* 2011; **52**: 285–292.

5 Abrahamian FM, Talan DA, Moran GJ. Management of skin and soft-tissue infections in the emergency department. *Infect Dis Clin North Am* 2008; **22**(1): 89–116, vi.

6 McConeghy KW, Mikolich DJ, LaPlante KL. Agents for the decolonization of methicillin-resistant Staphylococcus aureus. *Pharmacotherapy* 2009; **29**(3): 263–280.

7 Robicsek A, Beaumont JL, Thomson RB Jr, *et al.* Topical therapy for methicillin-resistant Staphylococcus aureus colonization: impact on infection risk. *Infect Control Hosp Epidemiol* 2009; **30**(7): 623–632.

8 AK. Skin and soft tissue infections. *Surg Clin North Am* 2009; **89**(2): 403–420, viii.

9 CE Rabuka, LY Azoulay, SR Kahn. Predictors of a positive duplex scan in patients with a clinical presentation compatible with deep vein thrombosis or cellulitis. *Can J Infect Dis* 2003; **14**(4): 210–214.

10 Bersier D, Bounameaux H. Cellulitis and deep vein thrombosis: a controversial association. *J Thromb Haemost* 2003; **1**(4): 867–868.

11 Arnold SR, Straus SE. Interventions to improve antibiotic prescribing practices in ambulatory care. *Cochrane Database Syst Rev* 2005; **4**: CD003539.

12 Gonzales R, Bartlett JG, Besser RE, *et al.* Principles of appropriate antibiotic use for treatment of uncomplicated acute bronchitis: background. *Ann Emerg Med* 2001; **37**(6): 720–727.

13 Centor RM, Witherspoon JM, Dalton HP, Brody CE, Link K. The diagnosis of strep throat in adults in the emergency room. *Med Decis Making* 1981; **1**: 239–246.

14 Cooper RJ, Hoffman JR, Bartlett JG, *et al.* Principles of appropriate antibiotic use for acute pharyngitis in adults: background. *Ann Emerg Med* 2001; **37**(6): 711–719.

15 Wing A, Villa-Roel C, Yeh B, Eskin B, Buckingham J, Rowe BH. Effectiveness of corticosteroid treatment in acute pharyngitis: a systematic review of the literature. *Acad Emerg Med* 2010; **17**(5): 476–483.

16 Hickner JM, Bartlett JG, Besser RE, *et al.* Principles of appropriate antibiotic use for acute rhinosinusitis in adults: background. *Ann Emerg Med* 2001; **37**(6): 703–710.

17 Gonzales R, Bartlett JG, Besser RE, *et al.* Principles of appropriate antibiotic use for treatment of acute respiratory tract infections in adults: background, specific aims, and methods. *Ann Emerg Med* 2001; **37**(6): 690–697.

18 Salkind AR. Clostridium difficile: an update for the primary care clinician. *South Med J* 2010; **103**(9): 896–902.

19 Pituch H. Clostridium difficile is no longer just a nosocomial infection or an infection of adults. *Int J Antimicrob Agents* 2009; **33** Suppl 1: S42–S45.

20 Bauer MP, van Dissel JT, Kuijper EJ. Clostridium difficile: controversies and approaches to management. *Curr Opin Infect Dis* 2009; **22**(6): 517–524.

21 Kuijper EJ, van Dissel JT, Wilcox MH. Clostridium difficile: changing epidemiology and new treatment options. *Curr Opin Infect Dis* 2007; **20**(4): 376–383.

22 Richards D, Toop L, Chambers S, Fletcher L. Response to antibiotics of women with symptoms of urinary tract infection but negative dipstick urine test results: double blind randomised controlled trial. *BMJ* 2005; **331**(7509): 143.

23 Cestari TF, Martignago BF. Scabies, pediculosis, bedbugs, and stinkbugs: uncommon presentations. *Clin Dermatol* 2005; **23**(6): 545–554.

24 Murray TS, Shapiro ED. Lyme disease. *Clin Lab Med* 2010; **30**(1): 311–328.

25 Nadelman RB, Nowakowski J, Fish D, *et al.* Prophylaxis with single-dose doxycycline for the prevention of Lyme disease after an Ixodes scapularis tick bite. *N Engl J Med* 2001; **345**(2): 79–84.

CHAPTER 9
Headache

Michael J. Laughlin Jr. and David M. Nestler
Department of Emergency Medicine, Mayo Clinic College of Medicine, Rochester, MN, USA

Introduction

Headaches are a common complaint in the emergent setting, and are responsible for 4% of all emergency department visits [1]. Nearly all patients with headache who present to an urgent care setting will have a benign cause and course. However, some causes of headache can be severe and life threatening. The practitioner must maintain a high level of suspicion when seeing a patient with a headache. One must be able to distinguish between a need for symptomatic relief in a patient with a routine headache, and the need for further diagnostic workup and management that may require a higher level of care.

Pitfall | **Failure to identify life-threatening headaches**

Classically, headaches are referred to as "primary" or "secondary" [2]. Primary headaches are those such as tension, migraine, or cluster headaches. These entities have a prevalence of 38%, 17%, and 0.4%, respectively [3–5]. Both migraine and tension-type headaches occur more in females, while cluster headaches are more common in men [6]. Migraine headaches are often unilateral, have gradual onset, are worse with activity, and cause patients to avoid light and sound [7]. Tension headaches are often bilateral, squeezing headaches, but allow the patient to perform his or her normal activities of daily living. Cluster headaches are characterized by unilateral, deep pain, associated with eye tearing and redness on the same side as the headache, a runny nose, and sweating. These primary headaches can be treated symptomatically and referred to primary care for follow up.

> KEY FACT | **Although headaches are common, sometimes they are secondary to serious pathology that may require complex diagnostics and management.**

Secondary headaches, however, are those attributable to other medical conditions. Although much less common than primary headaches, these headaches can be caused by infection, mass, or bleeding, to name a few causes (Box 9.1). These secondary headaches often require complex diagnostics, such as radiologic imaging, vital sign monitoring, and/or invasive procedures. It is therefore critical to differentiate primary from secondary headaches. Examples of critical secondary headaches are shown in Box 9.1.

Pitfall | **Failure to identify red flags for secondary headaches**

The keys to understanding who can be treated without diagnostic workup, and who needs immediate referral to a higher level of care, are the history and physical. A careful history and physical examination must be performed and documented on all headache patients. Headaches that are similar in nature and onset to prior episodes often can be treated symptomatically.

Urgent Care Emergencies: Avoiding the Pitfalls and Improving the Outcomes, First Edition.
Edited by Deepi G. Goyal and Amal Mattu.
© 2012 John Wiley & Sons, Ltd. Published 2012 by John Wiley & Sons, Ltd.

KEY FACT | **History and physical are the keys to understanding who requires aggressive diagnostic studies or management for their headaches.**

Box 9.1 Examples of causes of secondary headaches

Subarachnoid hemorrhage

Meningitis

Encephalitis

Cervico-cranial-artery dissection

Temporal arteritis

Acute angle-closure glaucoma

Hypertensive emergency

Carbon monoxide poisoning

Pseudotumor cerebri

Cerebral venous and dural sinus thrombosis

Acute stroke: either hemorrhagic or ischemic

Mass lesions including tumor, abscess, and hematoma

Source: Schenkel [20].

Some historical or physical examination features, however, can suggest a secondary headache requiring advanced care. The initial evaluation of headache should look for "red flags," which are historical or physical examination features that suggest a secondary cause of a headache [8]. Please see Box 9.2 for examples.

Pitfall | **If a patient has a history of headaches, they don't require any medical workup for this presentation**

Headaches are extremely common, and 94% of men and 99% of women report having a headache at some point in their life [6]. Headaches occur in different forms and different frequencies, but their ubiquitous prevalence should be noted. Therefore, it can be assumed that nearly every patient who presents for evaluation of a headache has suffered one in the past.

When population studies are reviewed and pooled, probabilities of different pathologies can be used to help to understand this issue further. One

---

Box 9.2 Historical or physical examination features that may suggest a serious secondary cause of headache

Worrisome features	Possible diagnosis
Rapid progression to maximal intensity over a matter of seconds	Intracranial bleeding or arterial dissection
"First-time" or "worst of life" headache	Intracranial hemorrhage or mass
Concomitant infection or immunosuppression	Intracranial infection
Acute visual changes, asymmetric eye findings, or abnormal funduscopic examination	Acute closed angle glaucoma, intracranial mass, temporal arteritis, or carotid artery dissection
Family history of subarachnoid hemorrhage	Subarachnoid hemorrhage
Headache spreading to lower neck	Intracranial hemorrhage or infection
Pain to palpation of the temple	Temporal arteritis
Similar headaches in people in close proximity	Exposure, such as carbon monoxide
Patient with history of cancer	Intracranial metastasis
Pregnant patient	Preeclampsia
Preceding head trauma or warfarin use	Intracranial hemorrhage
Significant hypertension	Intracranial hemorrhage or hypertensive encephalopathy
Confusion, altered mental status, or focal neurologic deficit	Intracranial mass, hemorrhage, or infection

systematic review reported that, before considering any other historical or physical examination features, the pretest probability of intracranial pathology for patients with chronic headache is about 1% [8]. However, this probability can increase to 43% if a history of thunderclap headache, or one that reaches maximal intensity in seconds, is reported. This data emphasizes the importance of history and physical examination. Consideration of "red flags" for a secondary cause of the particular headache in question remains the goal of the initial evaluation. Simply noting that the patient has suffered a headache in the past does not rule out secondary causes.

> KEY FACT | **Headaches are nearly ubiquitous in the population, and a history of prior headaches does not rule out worrisome secondary causes of the current headache in question.**

We must stress that not all patients who present with headache need to have a workup for a secondary cause. The key is to ask specific questions of every patient with headache to search for secondary causes. These would include questions about onset and rapidity of symptoms, "worst headache of life," or recent trauma (intracranial hemorrhage or vascular emergency), if there are family members, friends, or coworkers with headaches (carbon monoxide poisoning), visual changes (mass, ocular cause, temporal arteritis), anticoagulant use (intracranial hemorrhage), fever, rash, or neck pain (intracranial infection or vascular emergency), and immunosuppression (intracranial infection).

If major secondary causes for headache can be reasonably ruled out by history and physical examination, then it is likely that the patient does not need further testing.

Pitfall | **Assuming that a headache is benign because it responds to treatment**

When faced with a potential secondary cause of a headache, it may be tempting to treat the headache with medications first, and see how the patient responds. If a patient's headache improves with symptomatic treatment, however, this cannot be used to rule out secondary causes. Although there are no prospective randomized trials looking at this, there are numerous case reports where pain has significantly improved with symptomatic treatment, but the headache itself was caused by secondary pathology [9]. Response to triptans, anti-inflammatories, or analgesics can occur with any cause of headache, primary or secondary, and must not be used to exclude serious etiology. Although pain control is extremely important in the care of patients, the resolution of pain does not replace the need for ruling out life-threatening secondary causes of a headache.

> KEY FACT | **Response to symptomatic treatment does not rule out secondary causes of headache.**

Pitfall | **Relying on head CT to rule out serious causes of headache**

Head CTs are commonly performed in patients with headache. Although there is limited data on the number of patients presenting to the ED with headache, one Emergency Department study found that 1 out of every 14 ED patients received a head CT and, of those, 13% had presented with headache [10]. Although the full discussion is outside the scope of this review, practitioners must be judicious in ordering head CT scans, due to the cost and radiation exposure.

In patients with a reasonable concern for a serious secondary cause of their headache, however, the CT is often used. CTs can certainly be helpful in evaluating patients for intracranial structural abnormalities. The practitioner, however, also needs to remember that many serious secondary causes of headache can be present, even with a "negative" head CT (see Box 9.3).

The classic example where CT can be falsely reassuring is in patients with suspicion for subarachnoid hemorrhage (SAH). Computed tomography (CT) has excellent diagnostic capabilities, but is not infallible in missing SAH and other serious diagnoses. CT scans

Box 9.3 Secondary causes of headache often associated with a "negative" head CT

Subarachnoid hemorrhage

Increased intracranial pressure

Intracranial infection

Stroke

Arterial dissection

Hypertensive encephalopathy

Glaucoma

Temporal arteritis

Carbon monoxide poisoning

Preeclampsia

can miss small hemorrhages that are obscured by artifact or bone [9]. False negative CT scans, or those read incorrectly as "normal" in the setting of SAH, have been attributed to timing of the scan as well. The scan may not reveal acute bleeding if it began within a few hours of imaging, or if it occurred greater than one day prior to imaging [11]. In one report, amongst cases of confirmed SAH, CT scans performed five days after the hemorrhage identified acute blood in only 50% of the cases. Therefore, the lumbar puncture, with detection of blood in the sample, remains the "gold standard" for definitively ruling out SAH. If there is clinical concern for SAH, a patient needs to be evaluated in a setting where CT and lumbar puncture can be performed.

KEY FACT | **Patients with a history suggestive of subarachnoid hemorrhage should have a lumbar puncture if the head CT is normal.**

Pitfall | **Failure to consider CNS infection in the afebrile patient**

In the acute care setting, all patients who present with headache must have intracranial infection (meningitis or meningoencephalitis) in the differential diagnosis. Meningitis is rare, but potentially lethal. Providers must be vigilant, and obtain a thorough history and physical examination to safely exclude the diagnosis.

The classic triad of meningitis is (1) fever, (2) stiff neck, and (3) mental status changes. When these symptoms are observed, the diagnosis is virtually confirmed, and the patient would require transfer to a higher level of care, along with intravenous antibiotics or antivirals, consideration of steroids, and possible hospital admission for further care. However, the triad is only observed in 44% of adult patients with confirmed bacterial meningitis [12]. The most common symptom in meningitis is headache (87% of patients), followed by neck stiffness (83%), fever (77%), and mental status changes (69%). Therefore, approximately one in four patients with confirmed bacterial meningitis will NOT have a fever at presentation. Atypical presentations can be even more frequent in patients who are elderly or immunocompromised, or in patients with viral meningitis (i.e. herpes), and a heightened level of suspicion for meningitis must be maintained when evaluating these patients.

Treatment for the many causes of meningitis is beyond the scope of this book; however, if there is suspicion for bacterial meningitis, the patient should have broad-spectrum intravenous antibiotics initiated rapidly, even in the urgent care setting if possible. Emergent transfer to a higher-level institution is also warranted. At the receiving facility, further diagnostics, including imaging and lumbar puncture, can be performed and interpreted. It is commonplace to initiate antibiotics as soon as meningitis is suspected and before the lumbar puncture is performed. These antibiotics can be stopped if the results rule out meningitis. However, prompt initiation of treatment is always warranted.

KEY FACT | **Patients with CNS infections may be afebrile.**

Pitfall | **Failure to consider eclampsia in the pregnant patient**

Ironically, most pregnant women with a history of migraine headaches report that their migraines actually *improve* during the pregnancy. However, many patients will report headaches during their pregnancy, and although this can often be attributed to hormonal changes that occur, two diagnoses not to be missed in pregnant patients are stroke and preeclampsia.

Stroke appears to be more common in patients who are pregnant or have recently given birth [13]. While in the general population, thromboembolic strokes are much more common than hemorrhagic strokes, during pregnancy the incidence is equivalent. Eclampsia is considered to be the main cause of both thromboembolic and hemorrhagic strokes during and immediately after pregnancy.

Preeclampsia is defined as hypertension and proteinuria occurring after 20 weeks of gestation [14]. The cutoff for hypertension is either a systolic or diastolic blood pressure greater than 140/90, and proteinuria is at least 2+ on a dipstick. When seizures occur in the setting of preeclampsia, the patient is diagnosed as having eclampsia. Preeclampsia occurs in approximately 7% of pregnancies, and can occur any time during the pregnancy, or up to 12 weeks after delivery.

Taking a complete history is key in these patients who present with headache. Please see Box 9.4 for historical features that place a patient at higher risk for developing preeclampsia. If the acute care practitioner encounters a pregnant patient with a headache, they must pay particular attention to the blood pressure and the presence of edema on the physical examination. A blood pressure reading of 140/90 mm Hg or higher should prompt further evaluation for preeclampsia. Treatment for preeclampsia includes aggressive blood pressure control. Definitive therapy requires delivery of the fetus. Therefore, when this condition is suspected, further evaluation should be performed at a center capable of intravenous medication administration, aggressive blood pressure monitoring, and the capability for delivery.

> KEY FACT | **One must always consider preeclampsia in pregnant patients presenting with headaches.**

Pitfall | **Failure to identify carbon monoxide as a cause for headache**

Patients presenting for headache in the acute care setting often complain of associated symptoms. Aside from the headache, common symptoms include nausea (and possibly vomiting), fatigue, visual complaints, intolerance to noise, etc. A vital question to ask in the review of symptoms is, "Does anyone around you have similar symptoms?" Others in the household with headaches, nausea, and other symptoms can lead to the diagnosis of carbon monoxide (CO) poisoning.

Although rare, CO poisoning is a diagnosis not to be missed by the acute care practitioner. This can be potentially life-saving not only for the patient, but also for other household members or coworkers. CO poisoning results in approximately 500 unintentional deaths per year in the US [15]. Headache is the most common symptom in patients with CO poisoning [16] although, typically, there will be other nonspecific symptoms. Another key element in the review of systems is loss of consciousness (LOC). If a patient presents with a headache, LOC, and other household members are also ill, he or she needs to be referred to the nearest ED for further evaluation. Suspected CO poisoning must be evaluated by blood gas testing to measure the carboxyhemoglobin level. If the patient is referred, it is essential that the receiving facility is aware of the suspected diagnosis. If confirmed, treatment with hyperbaric oxygen therapy may be indicated.

> KEY FACT | **Clusters of headaches, or those related to specific environments, should prompt consideration of a toxin such as carbon monoxide.**

Box 9.4 Risk factors for preeclampsia

First pregnancy

Extremes of maternal age

History of hypertension

History of diabetes

Previous personal or family history of preeclampsia

Obesity

Multiple-gestation pregnancy

Concomitant visual changes

Concomitant abdominal pain

Pitfall | **Failure to identify headaches associated with increased intracerebral pressure**

seudotumor cerebri, also known as idiopathic intracranial hypertension (IIH), is defined by signs and symptoms related to elevated intracranial pressure. These include headache, papilledema, vision loss, diplopia, and pain behind the eyes. The most common symptom is headache (92% of patients) [17].

The headaches of IIH are nonspecific. Although their presentations vary widely, they are often described as quite severe, throbbing in nature, and related to position. The review of systems will be key in this diagnosis, as patients will frequently have visual complaints along with their headache. These can be transient visual obscurations, lasting just a few seconds at a time, or diplopia. Patients with a severe headache and new visual symptoms should raise concern for possible IIH.

A thorough physical examination should be performed, as the hallmark sign of IIH is papilledema. Interestingly, although the papilledema is typically bilateral, patients will often complain only of unilateral visual changes since the papilledema can be worse in one eye than in the other.

If the acute care practitioner is considering IIH, then brain imaging and possible lumbar puncture with opening pressure measurement is necessary. There is no pathognomonic feature of IIH on neuroimaging, but it is necessary not only in helping to diagnose IIH, but to exclude other causes of the patient's symptoms, especially in the setting of papilledema. These would include tumor, abscess, SAH, obstructive hydrocephalus, and venous sinus thrombosis, among many others. MRI is the preferred imaging modality, but CT is acceptable if there is no access to MRI. Clearly, if neuroimaging and/or lumbar puncture are not available at one's particular institution, a transfer to a higher level of care where these can be performed should occur, since undiagnosed IIH can lead to permanent visual loss.

KEY FACT | **Delayed diagnosis of pseudotumor cerebri can lead to permanent vision loss.**

Pitfall | **I do not see evidence of intracranial abnormality on history or physical examination, so I have ruled out all secondary causes**

Many extracranial secondary causes for headaches exist. Temporal arteritis (TA), also called giant cell arteritis, is a systemic vasculitis involving medium-sized arteries in the carotid circulation. One of the most common symptoms of TA is headache, while the most feared complication is visual loss. TA typically affects patients more than 50 years old, and is more common in women. The headache is typically localized to the temporal region of the face, and is described as "new" or different from any prior, potentially chronic headaches the patient may have experienced. Other symptoms include visual complaints such as partial or full blindness, jaw claudication, myalgias, fever, fatigue, and a history of polymyalgia rheumatica. Signs on examination include a prominent or thickened temporal artery, absent temporal pulse, and temporal artery tenderness [18]. A thorough eye examination and the serum measurement of erythrocyte sedimentation rate (ESR) are warranted in these patients. The ultimate diagnosis is made by temporal artery biopsy. It should be noted that patients often have an elevated ESR, but up to 20% of patients with biopsy-proven TA have normal ESR levels [19]. Treatment should be initiated by giving 40–60 mg per day of prednisone, and urgent biopsy of the temporal artery should be arranged.

Acute angle-closure glaucoma is another significant extracranial cause of headache. This is the most dangerous type of glaucoma since, if left untreated, it can lead to permanent visual loss in the affected eye. Headache is a common symptom in this disease. Other symptoms include eye pain or "cloudiness," nausea, vomiting, and abdominal pain.

If one suspects acute angle-closure glaucoma, then physical examination is of primary importance. Visual acuity must be performed, along with the evaluation of visual fields. Pupils need to be assessed for size and reactivity, since the affected pupil is typically mid-dilated and fixed. Intraocular pressures must be measured, as they can be as high as 50 mm Hg, and are typically above 20 mm Hg, in the affected eye. Lastly, a funduscopic examination should be performed.

The acute care practitioner must have a high level of suspicion for this disease entity, initiate treatment or transfer for treatment, and recommend emergent consultation from ophthalmology. If an ophthalmologist is unable to see the patient within an hour of diagnosis, treatment should be initiated. Treatment regimens may be practitioner dependent, but we recommend a topical β-blocker, a topical α-agonist, a topical steroid, and oral acetazolamide. Intraocular pressure in the affected eye must be assessed every 30 minutes to evaluate treatment efficacy. Whether this can be achieved in the acute care facility where the reader is practicing will be institution specific. The definitive treatment is iridotomy (creating a hole in the peripheral iris), performed by the ophthalmologist.

Another consideration for possible extracranial cause of secondary headache is toxicity. Recent medication changes, withdrawal from chronic medications or recreational substances, or exposures to carbon monoxide for example, have all been implicated as causing headaches. A careful social history, along with defining the events leading up to the onset of the headache, may be useful to identify extracranial causes.

> KEY FACT | **There are serious extracranial secondary causes for headache, including temporal arteritis, acute-angle closure glaucoma, and exposures. History and physical examination remain the mainstay for identifying these causes.**

Pearls to improve patient outcomes

- Although headaches are common, sometimes they are secondary to serious pathology that may require complex diagnostics and management.
- History and physical are the keys to understanding who requires aggressive diagnostic studies or management for their headaches.
- Headaches are nearly ubiquitous in the population, and a history of prior headaches does not rule out worrisome secondary causes of the current headache in question.

- Response to symptomatic treatment does not rule out secondary causes of headache.
- Patients with a history suggestive of subarachnoid hemorrhage should have a lumbar puncture if the head CT is normal.
- Patients with CNS infections may be afebrile.
- One must always consider preeclampsia in pregnant patients presenting with headaches.
- Clusters of headaches, or those related to specific environments, should prompt consideration of a toxin such as carbon monoxide.
- Delayed diagnosis of pseudotumor cerebri can lead to permanent vision loss.
- There are serious extracranial secondary causes for headache, including temporal arteritis, acute-angle closure glaucoma, and exposures. History and physical examination remain the mainstay for identifying these causes.

References

1 Ramirez-Lassepas M, Espinosa CE, Cicero JJ, *et al.* Predictors of intracranial pathologic findings in patients who seek emergency care because of headache. *Arch Neurol* 1997; **54**(12): 1506–1509.

2 Headache Classification Subcommittee of the International Headache Society. The International Classification of Headache Disorders: 2nd edition. *Cephalalgia* 2004; **24**(Suppl 1): 9–160.

3 Schwartz BS, Stewart WF, Simon D, Lipton RB. Epidemiology of tension-type headache. *JAMA* 1998; **279**(5): 381–383.

4 Sjaastad O, Bakketeig LS. Cluster headache prevalence. Vågå study of headache epidemiology. *Cephalalgia* 2003; **23**(7): 528–533.

5 Stewart WF, Shechter A, Rasmussen BK. Migraine prevalence. A review of population-based studies. *Neurology* 1994; **44**(6 Suppl 4): S17–S23.

6 Rasmussen BK, Jensen R, Schroll M, Olesen J. Epidemiology of headache in a general population – a prevalence study. *J Clin Epidemiol* 1991; **44**(11): 1147–1157.

7 Cutrer F. Evaluation of the adult patient with headache in the emergency department. *UpToDate.com* 2010.

8 Detsky ME, McDonald DR, Baerlocher MO, *et al.* Does this patient with headache have a migraine or need neuroimaging? *JAMA* 2006; **296**(10): 1274–1283.

9 Edlow JA, Panagos PD, Godwin SA, *et al*. Clinical policy: critical issues in the evaluation and management of adult patients presenting to the emergency department with acute headache. *Ann Emerg Med.* 2008; **52**(4): 407–436.

10 Raja AS, Andruchow J, Zane R, Khorasani R, Schuur JD. Use of neuroimaging in US emergency departments. *Arch Intern Med* 2011; **171**(3): 260–262.

11 Kassell NF, Torner JC, Haley EC, *et al*. The International Cooperative Study on the Timing of Aneurysm Surgery. Part 1: Overall management results. *J Neurosurg* 1990; **73**(1): 18–36.

12 Van de Beek D, de Gans J, Spanjaard L, *et al*. Clinical features and prognostic factors in adults with bacterial meningitis. *N Engl J Med* 2004; **351**(18): 1849–1859.

13 Sharshar T, Lamy C, Mas JL. Incidence and causes of strokes associated with pregnancy and puerperium. A study in public hospitals of Ile de France. Stroke in Pregnancy Study Group. *Stroke* 1995; **26**(6): 930–936.

14 Lipstein H, Lee CC, Crupi RS. A current concept of eclampsia. *Am J Emerg Med* 2003; **21**(3): 223–226.

15 Centers for Disease Control and Prevention (CDC). Unintentional non-fire-related carbon monoxide exposures – United States, 2001–2003. *Morb Mortal Wkly Rep* 2005; **54**(2): 36–39.

16 Tomaszewski C. Carbon monoxide poisoning. Early awareness and intervention can save lives. *Postgrad Med* 1999; **105**(1): 39–40, 3–8, 50.

17 Wall M, George D. Idiopathic intracranial hypertension. A prospective study of 50 patients. *Brain* 1991; **114**(Pt 1A): 155–180.

18 Smetana GW, Shmerling RH. Does this patient have temporal arteritis? *JAMA* 2002; **287**(1): 92–101.

19 Villa-Forte A. Giant cell arteritis: suspect it, treat it promptly. *Cleve Clin J Med* 2011; **78**(4): 265–270.

20 Schenkel S. Chapter Title: Headache Management. In: Mattu A, Goyal D (eds.), *Emergency Medicine: Avoiding the Pitfalls and Improving the Outcomes* (1st edn.). Blackwell Publishing, Massachusetts; 2007: p. 42.

CHAPTER 10

The Evaluation and Management of Back Pain

Michael C. Bond

Department of Emergency Medicine, University of Maryland School of Medicine, Baltimore, MD, USA

Introduction

Back pain is an extremely common complaint among patients presenting to urgent care centers and emergency departments (EDs). In 2007, back problems were reported by 27 million adults aged 18 and older in the United States; more than 19.1 million received treatment for back pain, with a direct cost of $30.3 billion [1]. The annual direct care cost for back pain is estimated to be $12.2 to $90.6 billion in the United States [2]. These figures do not include the indirect costs of lost work days or disability payments, estimated to be $7.4 to $28.2 billion per year [3]. In 2005, the estimated mean age- and sex-adjusted medical expenditure among respondents with spine problems was $6,096 versus $3,516 for those without spine problems in 2005 [4].

Pitfall | Failure to recognize the "red flags" in the medical history or physical exam that suggest a serious cause of a patient's back pain

Most cases of back pain do not have a discernible cause, but they have a predictable course. A subset of patients is at risk for chronic pain and disability, and in another subset, a serious life-threatening or devastating neurologic disease will develop if appropriate treatment is not administered. Identifying the patients at risk for an underlying disease is paramount in the evaluation of back pain. Given the frequency with which musculoskeletal back pain is seen in the acute care setting, it is easy to become complacent with the evaluation. This is most likely to occur when evaluating patients who have a history of chronic back pain, as an acute exacerbation of the pain is the most likely cause of their presentation; however, a more serious disease could be present. The evaluation of all patients with back pain should include a comprehensive history and physical exam. Describing how to conduct a complete physical examination is beyond the scope of this article, but key factors that should be documented are highlighted below. The history should specifically cover the "red flags" in Box 10.1. Patients with any of these signs and symptoms should undergo additional diagnostic testing as indicated.

All patients should be undressed for the examination. This allows direct visualization of rashes (e.g. herpes zoster); asymmetric muscle development or atrophy; scars that indicate previous surgical repairs or trauma; and evidence of recent trauma, such as lacerations, abrasions, or ecchymosis. It also permits a more thorough sensory exam and examination of the lower back. The physical examination should consist of formal and functional strength testing.

Urgent Care Emergencies: Avoiding the Pitfalls and Improving the Outcomes, First Edition.

Edited by Deepi G. Goyal and Amal Mattu.

© 2012 John Wiley & Sons, Ltd. Published 2012 by John Wiley & Sons, Ltd.

Box 10.1 Red flags in patient history and physical examination

Red flags: history	Red flags: physical
• Age <18 or >50 years old • Pain lasting more than 6 weeks • History of cancer • Fever • Night sweats • Unexplained weight loss • Recent bacterial infection • Intravenous drug abuse • Immunocompromised state (e.g. HIV infection, immunosuppression) • Major trauma • Minor trauma in the elderly • Night pain or pain that increases when supine	• Fever • Bowel or bladder incontinence • Saddle anesthesia • Decreased or absent anal sphincter tone • New neurologic deficit

Formal testing typically consists of the patient resisting against the examiner and is graded on a scale of 1 to 5. However, because of pain, many patients are unable or unwilling to cooperate fully with strength testing. Having patients walk or lift up on their toes, rock back on their heels, and squat allows evaluation of the strength in their quadriceps, hamstrings, and dorsiflexors. If the patient is unable to raise one leg, the examiner should note whether the patient is pushing down with the other leg. If no contralateral effort is being exerted (i.e. the patient is not pushing down), then the patient either is not fully cooperating with the examination or has bilateral leg weakness.

The patient's gait should be observed. Ideally, when possible, the examiner should observe the patient's gait as he or she walks to the examination room. It is not unusual for the gait to be slower and less natural when patients know they are being observed. Special attention should be directed toward ensuring the patient does not have foot drop, is not dragging a leg, and has a normal swing phase of the gait when all the weight is on a single

leg. With the patient in a standing position, his or her range of motion in anterior flexion, posterior flexion, and lateral flexion should be assessed.

If the patient complains of urinary or stool incontinence, or if the physical examination yields findings indicative of incontinence, a rectal examination checking sphincter tone should be performed. If the patient has urinary incontinence, a bladder scan should be requested or the post-void residual should be measured to exclude a neurogenic bladder. Incontinence can be caused by overflow incontinency from the inability to drain the bladder completely.

Pediatric back pain

Historically, it has been taught that back pain in children and adolescents is rare; however, the true incidence is not known, as many children with this pain do not seek medical care. Recent literature suggests that a relatively high number of children do experience back pain [5]. As in adults, an identifiable cause of the pain often is not evident. Davis *et al.* modified the traditional red flags (Box 10.2) to address the specific disease processes that can occur in the pediatric population [5]. The physical examination in the child is similar to that in adults, though special care should be taken to look for scoliosis and kyphosis. A lower extremity examination is also needed to ensure that the child is not experiencing referred pain from the knee or hip.

KEY FACT | **Recent literature suggests that a relatively high number of children do experience back pain. As in adults, an identifiable cause of the pain often is not evident.**

As in adults, children should have an assessment of their forward flexion. Schober's measurement is obtained by placing a mark 10 cm above and 5 cm below the level of the sacral dimples. This distance is measured, and the patient is then asked to touch his or her toes. The distance between the marks is measured again at the patient's maximum reach. A problem with lumbar mobility is suggested if the distance between the marks does not increase by

---

Box 10.2 Historical and physical examination red flags in children

Red flags: history	Red flags: physical
• Prepubertal children, especially <5 years • Functional disability • Duration >4 weeks • Recurrent or worsening pain • Early morning stiffness and/or gelling • Night pain • Fever, weight loss, malaise • Postural changes: kyphosis or scoliosis • Limp or altered gait	• Fever, tachycardia • Weight loss, bruising, lymphadenopathy, or abdominal mass • Altered spine shape or mobility • Vertebral or intervertebral tenderness • Limp or altered gait • Neurologic symptoms • Bladder or bowel dysfunction

Reproduced from Davis and Williams [5] with permission from the BMJ Publishing Group.

---

more than 7 cm. Children with scoliosis should have a determination of whether it is fixed or reversible. Fixed scoliosis does not change with movements and is caused by a structural anomaly. Reversible scoliosis is typically related to posture or an abnormality of the pelvis or leg (e.g. a leg length discrepancy).

Evaluation

There is no standard evaluation that is required in patients with back pain. In the vast majority of cases, regardless of the patient's age, laboratory studies (e.g. complete blood count (CBC), urinalysis (UA), blood cultures (BCx), C-reactive protein (CRP), and elevated sedimentation rate (ESR)), radiographs, and magnetic resonance imaging (MRI) do not alter the management of the patient and only increase the cost of care. Radiographs should be ordered in cases of trauma, for the elderly when there is concern for compression fractures or cancer, and for children in whom a congenital anomaly or occult trauma may be present. MRI scans often identify pathology that may not be responsible for the patient's pain. In a study by Jensen *et al.*, 52% of completely asymptomatic individuals had at least one herniated nucleus pulposus (HNP) on MRI [6]. Similar findings have been found in other studies, so it has become clear that HNPs are often found but are not necessarily the cause of the patient's back pain. In fact, MRI is best used to determine if the HNP is compressing any neural structures. MRI is the preferred test if there is concern for cancer, infection, disk pathology, or spinal stenosis. Computed tomography (CT) scans are better for bony detail and are preferred if a fracture is suspected.

> KEY FACT | **In the vast majority of cases, laboratory studies and imaging do not alter the management and only increase the cost of care.**

Treatment

The treatment of low back pain should be aimed at returning the patient to work and usual activity level as quickly as possible. Most patients improve within 6 weeks regardless of the treatment rendered. Patients should be encouraged to return to light activity. Bed rest should be discouraged. A recent Cochrane review revealed moderate evidence that patients experience pain relief and a return to functional status when they stay active.

> KEY FACT | **Most patients improve within 6 weeks regardless of the treatment rendered.**

The preferred drugs for pain control are nonsteroidal anti-inflammatory drugs (NSAIDs) and acetaminophen, which have been shown to be as effective as muscle relaxants and opiates [7, 8]. Opiates and muscle relaxants are associated with more severe side effects and should be used only when absolutely needed, and then for the shortest time possible. However, a recent analysis of the National Hospital Ambulatory Medical Care Survey showed that two thirds of ED patients who presented with back pain were prescribed opiates, which were prescribed more often than NSAIDs [9]. There is no proven benefit to glucocorticosteroids in patients with back pain or sciatica [7]. They are not recommended because of their side effect profile, which includes an increased risk of infection, gastrointestinal bleeding, and hyperglycemia.

Exercise is one of the few treatment modalities shown to be effective for chronic low back pain [10]. Patients with chronic pain and those who are not responding to conservative therapy should be referred to physical therapy. After 6 weeks of conservative treatment, and if physical therapy is ineffective, patients should be referred to a back pain specialist for further diagnostic tests (e.g. MRI), consideration for epidural corticosteroid injections, or surgery.

> KEY FACT | **Exercise is one of the few treatment modalities shown to be effective for chronic low back pain.**

Specific disease processes

Pitfall | **Failure to consider the diagnosis of spinal epidural abscess because the patient does not have a fever or neurologic deficit**

Epidural abscess

Spinal epidural abscesses (SEAs) are rare, with an estimated incidence of 1 in 10,000 hospital admissions. They have been increasing in frequency over the past 25 years. Risk factors for a spinal epidural abscess are listed in Box 10.3. The classic triad of fever, back pain, and neurologic deficit is seen in less than 15% of patients at the time of initial presentation, and only 50% of this group is febrile initially [11]. This makes the diagnosis of SEA

Box 10.3 Risk factors for spinal epidural abscess

Diabetes

End-stage renal disease

Septicemia

HIV infection

Malignancy

Morbid obesity

Long-term glucocorticoid use

Intravenous drug abuse

Alcoholism

Infection at a distal site

Indwelling catheters

History of spinal surgery

Source: Tompkins *et al.* [13].

challenging. Half of the cases of SEA are misdiagnosed on the initial visit. The diagnosis should be considered in patients with new onset of back pain and risk factors or with back pain associated with fever, chills, night sweats, weight loss, or any neurologic deficit. Unfortunately, laboratory tests alone cannot make the diagnosis. Neither the total white blood cell (WBC) count nor the leukocyte percentage is helpful in the diagnosis. Several studies have shown that the WBC count is greater than 12,000 cells/mm^3 in only 60% of cases [12]. CRP and ESR can be elevated but are not specific for SEA and are best used to follow the patient's response to therapy. Blood cultures are positive in only 60% of patients. Plain radiographs can visualize the very late signs associated with osteomyelitis or foreign bodies [13]. MRI with gadolinium is the only test that is sensitive and specific enough to make the diagnosis.

> KEY FACT | **The classic triad of fever, back pain, and neurologic deficit is seen in less than 15% of patients at the time of initial presentation, and only 50% of this group is febrile initially.**

The goal of early diagnosis and treatment is to prevent further neurologic injury. The mortality rate is still estimated to be 10% to 23% despite surgery and antibiotics. The most important prognostic indicator of the patient's final neurologic outcome is his or her preoperative neurologic function. Patients who present with a neurologic deficit are less likely to regain full function, and those who have had neurologic symptoms longer than 36 hours are unlikely to regain any function.

> KEY FACT | **The most important prognostic indicator of the patient's final neurologic outcome is his or her preoperative neurologic function.**

The fact that a patient is afebrile, has a normal neurologic examination, or has a normal WBC count should not dissuade the acute care provider from performing a more thorough evaluation with MRI if the pretest probability is moderate to high. Low-risk patients who are afebrile, have a normal exam, and have normal laboratory values can be discharged with close follow-up with their primary care provider.

If MRI and spine surgery capabilities are not immediately available, the acute care provider should immediately transfer any high-risk patient to a center that has these resources.

Vertebral osteomyelitis

Pitfall | **Starting antibiotics in patients in whom vertebral osteomyelitis is suspected but who have normal neurologic exams**

The presentation of vertebral osteomyelitis can be similar to that of SEA. The risk factors and the causative organisms for osteomyelitis are the same as those for SEA. Elderly patients and those who have had recent surgery or urinary tract infections are at risk for infection with gram-negative organisms. Patients typically present with chronic back pain that has developed gradually over weeks and months. As in SEA, laboratory values (e.g. ESR, CRP, or WBC count) and plain radiographs cannot exclude the diagnosis and are not specific enough to confirm the diagnosis. MRI or CT is needed to confirm the diagnosis and will show abnormalities in 70% to 90% of patients with osteomyelitis [14].

Patients with osteomyelitis are treated with a 6- to 12-week course of antibiotics specific to the causative organism. In many cases, the organism must be identified from bone biopsy or operative sample; therefore, it is recommended that antibiotics not be started until appropriate samples can be obtained. Antibiotics should not be withheld from patients who have a neurologic deficit on presentation.

The acute care provider should obtain an MRI or CT scan emergently when the diagnosis is suspected and refer the patient to an appropriate spine surgeon if the diagnosis is confirmed. Short-term treatment consists of analgesics, with antibiotics being held until the case can be discussed with a spine surgeon.

> KEY FACT | **In many cases, the organism must be identified from bone biopsy or operative sample; therefore, it is recommended that antibiotics not be started until appropriate samples can be obtained.**

Spinal cord compression

Pitfall | **Failure to consider spinal cord compression in patients who experience an increase in back pain when they are recumbent**

Spinal cord compression (SCC) is a true medical emergency that has a multitude of causes, including HNPs, cancer (primary or metastatic), epidural hematomas, epidural abscesses, and displaced vertebral fractures. The most common cause is a massive midline disc herniation, usually at the L4–L5 level [12]. Though the causes of SCC can vary, a consistent characteristic is that patients present with back pain that is worse with recumbency and ultimately associated with progressive neurologic deficits. Patients will go on to develop a bilateral or unilateral radiculopathy, followed by sensory deficits with symmetric and bilateral weakness. Saddle anesthesia with bowel, bladder, or erectile dysfunction is a late finding. Patients may also develop urinary incontinence due to overflow incontinency secondary to a neurogenic bladder.

KEY FACT | **Though the causes can vary, a consistent characteristic is that patients present with back pain that is worse with recumbency and ultimately associated with progressive neurologic deficits.**

The primary determinant of the patient's ultimate neurologic status is his or her status at the time of diagnosis. Therefore, it is imperative that the diagnosis be made early, prior to the development of any neurologic deficit. In fact, a normal neurologic examination should not exclude the diagnosis if the pretest probability of the presence of SCC is moderate to high. Unfortunately, laboratory studies cannot exclude the diagnosis. The diagnosis can be excluded only with MRI or, for those who cannot tolerate the MRI process, with CT myelography.

The acute care provider should suspect SCC when patients complain of back pain that is worse when they are supine and is relieved when they sit up; if the patient has any neurologic deficits; if the patient has history of cancer or a HNP; or if risk factors for epidural hematoma (i.e. the patient is taking anticoagulants) or epidural abscess (see previous section) are present.

The ultimate treatment (e.g. surgery for a hematoma or abscess or radiation for cancer) will be dictated by the cause, but all patients can benefit from high-dose glucocorticoids.

Glucocorticoids minimize ongoing neurologic damage caused by compression by decreasing the edema in the spinal cord. Dosing varies and remains controversial, but dexamethasone, 10 to 100 mg, administered intravenously has been recommended. Higher dose steroids are associated with more side effects (e.g. infection and hyperglycemia) but have better evidence for improving neurologic outcomes. There are no good randomized studies assessing neurologic outcomes following administration of low-dose glucocorticoids [15].

KEY FACT | **The ultimate treatment (e.g. surgery for a hematoma or abscess or radiation for cancer) will be dictated by the cause, but all patients can benefit from high-dose glucocorticoids.**

The acute care provider should start high-dose glucocorticoids and immediately transfer the patient to a center that has the capability to perform emergent MRI and that has a spine surgeon and radiation oncology services if they are not available at the initial location.

Abdominal aortic aneurysm

Pitfall | **Failure to consider the diagnosis of abdominal aortic aneurysm or aortic dissection in elderly patients with back pain**

Low back pain is a significant complaint in more than 30% of adults 65 years or older. Although the majority of cases have a benign cause, one must consider vascular causes. Abdominal aortic aneurysm (AAA) and aortic dissection (AD) cause 1% of the deaths in this age group, accounting for 15,000 deaths annually in the United States [16]. Though the abrupt onset of severe back pain increases the suspicion for AAA rupture or an acute dissection, patients with these conditions can experience a chronic onset of back pain. In one case series, patients with unruptured AAA experienced back pain from 1 to 60 days (mean, 11.6 days) before the diagnosis was made [17]. Making the correct diagnosis of AAA is further complicated by the fact that a pulsatile abdominal mass was noted in only 26% of patients who were misdiagnosed on their initial evaluation [18]. Other investigators have reported that the sensitivity of abdominal palpation in detecting a pulsatile mass is poor, reaching 80% only for aneurysms at least 5 cm in diameter [19–21].

KEY FACT | **Making the correct diagnosis of AAA is further complicated by the fact that a pulsatile abdominal mass was noted in only 26% of patients who were misdiagnosed on their initial evaluation.**

Isolated back pain is a relatively rare presentation of a ruptured AAA. Lloyd *et al.* reported that only 4% of patients had back pain as their sole chief complaint, whereas 14% of patients had both abdominal and back pain [22]. In the series described by Yoshioka *et al.*, 77.5% of patients with aortic dissection had at least some back pain, and 45% presented with sudden severe isolated back pain [23].

Clearly, not all elderly patients who present with low back pain need an evaluation for AAA or AD. However, the diagnosis of AAA or AD should be assumed in any patient who has back pain and syncope and should be strongly considered in hypertensive elderly patients with non-traumatic back pain of new onset.

Cancer

Pitfall | **Failure to consider a primary cancer or metastasis to the spine as a cause of back pain**

Cancer can metastasize to the spinal column and cause back pain. Pain can result from cancer growth within the epidural space (causing SCC), intramedullary growth within the vertebrae, or direct extension of the primary cancer into the vertebrae and spinal cord. Back pain is often the initial symptom of spinal metastasis and is often described as a constant dull pain that is not relieved with rest; it may increase with recumbency. The neurologic signs and symptoms associated with SCC (see above) are not uncommon.

If the patient has no neurologic deficits, the initial evaluation can consist of plain radiographs, which may show destructive bony lesions. If destructive lesions are present and the patient has no neurologic deficits, it is acceptable to schedule an MRI scan within 24 hours to more thoroughly evaluate the lesions. In all other cases, MRI is the imaging modality of choice and should be done emergently. As for SCC, glucocorticosteroids are recommended to reduce spinal cord edema in patients with neurologic deficits. Typically, MRI scans are limited to the area in which the patient is having pain; however, in patients with cancer, an entire spine MRI scan should be obtained, since they are at risk for metastasis at multiple levels and some lesions might not be symptomatic on the initial presentation.

If MRI and oncology services are not available in the facility where the patient is seen initially, the acute care provider should consider transferring patients with cancer and back pain to a center with those resources.

Spinal compression fractures

Osteoporosis in the elderly can lead to spinal compression fractures without any preceding trauma. These fractures are a major cause of chronic pain and disability, limiting a patient's ability to pursue his or her daily activities. It is important to consider malignancy as a cause of the fracture.

Plain radiographs of the back should be obtained to exclude spinal compression fractures in the evaluation of patients over 65 years of age who present with back pain. If a fracture is seen and cancer is suspected, the patient should also undergo high-resolution CT of the spine. High-resolution CT can distinguish between benign and malignant causes of vertebral compression fractures and is more readily available than MRI [24].

A simple compression fracture can be treated with analgesics (e.g. NSAIDs, acetaminophen, or narcotics) and supportive care. The acute care provider can also consider starting calcitonin, which has been shown to decrease the pain associated with compression fractures without the typical side effects seen with NSAIDs and narcotics [25]. Patients can be referred for vertebroplasty, which alleviates the pain of compression fractures, improves quality of life, and restores the vertebral column to its pre-fracture height [16].

KEY FACT | **Calcitonin has been shown to decrease the pain associated with compression fractures without the typical side effects seen with NSAIDs and narcotics.**

Spinal stenosis

Spinal stenosis is seen most commonly in the elderly with degenerative arthritis. Patients will typically complain of bilateral lower back pain that is worse with walking, prolonged standing, or spinal extension and relieved when the patient sits, lies down, or bends forward at the waist. Patients often complain of burning back pain that radiates to the buttocks and posterolateral legs when they are active. The symptoms are caused by stenosis of the vertebral canal, resulting from a combination of loss of intervertebral disc height, facet joint hypertrophy, and thickening of the ligament flavum. These changes cause a narrowing of the cross-sectional diameter of the spinal canal and neural foramina when the back is extended (i.e. when the patient is upright), which results in mechanical compression and nerve root ischemia.

Spinal stenosis can be diagnosed based on the history and physical examination alone. In the absence of any red flags, there is no need for any diagnostic testing to be done in the acute setting. Patients should be treated with NSAIDs or acetaminophen and can complete their evaluation on a non-urgent basis. MRI is the study of choice, though CT myelography can be performed in those who are claustrophobic or have a contraindication to a MRI scan (e.g. a pacemaker). Patients with a neurologic deficit should undergo MRI or CT myelography immediately.

Pregnancy-related low back pain

Back pain is experienced by 50% to 90% of women during pregnancy [27]. The risk factors for back pain during pregnancy are advanced maternal age, a history of back pain, and the number of pregnancies. Neither fetal weight nor the amount of weight gained by the mother is associated with an increased risk of back pain [28].

Pitfall | **Treating pregnancy-related back pain with NSAIDs**

The causes of back pain during pregnancy are multifactorial. Pregnant women are at risk for development of spondylolysis and progression of their underlying spondylolisthesis. In fact, parous woman have a higher incidence of L4–L5 spondylolisthesis than their nulliparous counterparts [29]. The majority of patients can be treated successfully with a support binder or acetaminophen. NSAIDs should be avoided in pregnancy because of the risk of premature closure of the patent ductus arteriosus, preterm birth, and fetal renal abnormalities. Narcotics can be used with no harm to the baby.

> KEY FACT | **Back pain is experienced by 50% to 90% of women during pregnancy.**

In patients whose pain is not relieved with conservative measures, imaging studies may be required. Plain radiographs and CT are generally avoided, as they expose the fetus to ionizing radiation. The fetus cannot be effectively shielded when obtaining lumbar spine radiographs. A MRI scan can be obtained and is completely safe in pregnancy; however, unless the mother is exhibiting neurologic deficits, it is unlikely that any findings will be acted on until after the baby is delivered. Therefore, reassurance, frequent examinations to confirm the absence of neurologic deficit, and pain control might be all that is needed to allow the patient to complete her pregnancy. If the pain does not resolve in the post-partum period, further diagnostic testing should be obtained.

Pearls for improving patient outcomes

• All patients with back pain must be assessed for the presence of "red flags" that are markers of a serious underlying disease.
• Refer patients with red flags in their history or on physical examination for a more comprehensive evaluation, which may include laboratory testing, radiographs, CT, or MRI.
• Do not assume that a herniated nucleus pulposus is the cause of an individual's back pain.
• Use acetaminophen and NSAIDs as first-line treatment for pain control in patients with back pain. Prescribe narcotics and muscle relaxants only when necessary and for the shortest duration possible.
• Exercise is one of the few treatment modalities to be proven effective in the treatment of back pain.
• Consider the diagnosis of spinal epidural abscess in patients with fever, neurologic deficits, or risk factors for spinal epidural abscess when they present with atraumatic back pain.
• Start high-dose glucocorticoids as soon as possible in patients with spinal cord compression.

• Consider aortic dissection and aortic aneurysm in hypertensive patients who present with sudden onset of atraumatic back pain.
• Consider starting calcitonin in patients with vertebral compression fractures.

References

1 Soni A. Statistical Brief #289, Back Problems: Use and Expenditures for the U.S. Adult Population, 2007. In: *MEPS: Medical Expenditure Panel Survey*. AHRQ: Agency for Healthcare Research and Quality; 2010.

2 Haldeman S, Dagenais S. A supermarket approach to the evidence-informed management of chronic low back pain. *Spine J* 2008; **8**: 1–7.

3 Dagenais S, Caro J, Haldeman S. A systematic review of low back pain cost of illness studies in the United States and internationally. *Spine J* 2008; **8**: 8–20.

4 Martin BI, Deyo RA, Mirza SK, *et al*. Expenditures and health status among adults with back and neck problems. *JAMA* 2008; **299**: 656–64.

5 Davis PJ, Williams HJ. The investigation and management of back pain in children. *Arch Dis Child Educ Pract Ed* 2008; **93**: 73–83.

6 Jensen MC, Brant-Zawadzki MN, Obuchowski N, *et al*. Magnetic resonance imaging of the lumbar spine in people without back pain. *N Engl J Med* 1994; **331**: 69–73.

7 Chou R, Huffman LH. Medications for acute and chronic low back pain: a review of the evidence for an American Pain Society/American College of Physicians clinical practice guideline. *Ann Intern Med* 2007; **147**: 505–514.

8 Chou R, Qaseem A, Snow V, *et al*. Diagnosis and treatment of low back pain: a joint clinical practice guideline from the American College of Physicians and the American Pain Society. *Ann Intern Med* 2007; **147**: 478–491.

9 Friedman BW, Chilstrom M, Bijur PE, *et al*. Diagnostic testing and treatment of low back pain in United States emergency departments: a national perspective. *Spine J* 2010; **35**: E1406–E1411.

10 Maher CG. Effective physical treatment for chronic low back pain. *Orthop Clin North Am* 2004; **35**: 57–64.

11 Darouiche RO. Spinal epidural abscess. *N Engl J Med* 2006; **355**: 2012–2020.

12 Corwell BN. The emergency department evaluation, management, and treatment of back pain. *Emerg Med Clin North Am* 2010; **28**: 811–839.

13 Tompkins M, Panuncialman I, Lucas P, *et al*. Spinal epidural abscess. *J Emerg Med* 2010; **39**: 384–390.

14 Beronius M, Bergman B, Andersson R. Vertebral osteomyelitis in Göteborg, Sweden: a retrospective study of patients during 1990–95. *Scand J Infect Dis* 2001; **33**: 527–532.

15 Loblaw DA, Laperriere NJ. Emergency treatment of malignant extradural spinal cord compression: an evidence-based guideline. *J Clin Oncol* 1998; **16**: 1613–1624.

16 Broder J, Snarski JT. Back pain in the elderly. *Clin Geriatr Med* 2007; **23**: 271–289.

17 Cambria RA, Gloviczki P, Stanson AW, *et al*. Symptomatic, nonruptured abdominal aortic aneurysms: are emergent operations necessary? *Ann Vasc Surg* 1994; **8**: 121–126.

18 Marston WA, Ahlquist R, Johnson G Jr, *et al*. Misdiagnosis of ruptured abdominal aortic aneurysms. *J Vasc Surg* 1992; **16**: 17–22.

19 Fink HA, Lederle FA, Roth CS, *et al*. The accuracy of physical examination to detect abdominal aortic aneurysm. *Arch Intern Med* 2000; **160**: 833–836.

20 Lederle FA, Simel DL. The rational clinical examination. Does this patient have abdominal aortic aneurysm? *JAMA* 1999; **281**: 77–82.

21 Venkatasubramaniam AK, Mehta T, Chetter IC, *et al*. The value of abdominal examination in the diagnosis of abdominal aortic aneurysm. *Eur J Vasc Endovasc Surg* 2004; **27**: 56–60.

22 Lloyd GM, Bown MJ, Norwood MG, *et al*. Feasibility of preoperative computer tomography in patients with ruptured abdominal aortic aneurysm: a time-to-death study in patients without operation. *J Vasc Surg* 2004; **39**: 788–791.

23 Yoshioka K, Toribatake Y, Kawahara N, *et al*. Acute aortic dissection or ruptured aortic aneurysm associated with back pain and paraplegia. *Orthopedics* 2008; **31**: 651.

24 Kubota T, Yamada K, Ito H, *et al*. High-resolution imaging of the spine using multidetector-row computed tomography: differentiation between benign and malignant vertebral compression fractures. *J Comput Assist Tomogr* 2005; **29**: 712–719.

25 Lyritis GP, Ioannidis GV, Karachalios T, *et al*. Analgesic effect of salmon calcitonin suppositories in patients with acute pain due to recent osteoporotic vertebral crush fractures: a prospective double-blind, randomized, placebo-controlled clinical study. *Clin J Pain* 1999; **15**: 284–289.

26 Hall S, Bartleson JD, Onofrio BM, *et al*. Lumbar spinal stenosis. Clinical features, diagnostic procedures, and

results of surgical treatment in 68 patients. *Ann Intern Med* 1985; **103**: 271–275.

27 Pivarnik JM, Chambliss HO, Clapp JF, *et al.* Impact of physical activity during pregnancy and postpartum on chronic disease risk. *Med Sci Sports Exerc* 2006; **38**: 989–1006.

28 Meleger AL, Krivickas LS. Neck and back pain: musculoskeletal disorders. *Neurol Clin* 2007; **25**: 419–438.

29 Sanderson PL, Fraser RD. The influence of pregnancy on the development of degenerative spondylolisthesis. *J Bone Joint Surg, Br Vol* 1996; **78**: 951–954.

CHAPTER 11
Pediatric Pitfalls

Jana L. Anderson and James L. Homme
Department of Emergency Medicine and Pediatrics, Mayo Clinic, Rochester, MN, USA

Introduction

Caring for children in the acute care setting poses many challenges. Physiologic differences from adults, early language development, and inherent apprehension of providers contribute to these challenges. Additionally, these challenges tempt the practitioner to either (a) over-diagnose certain common conditions such as acute otitis media as an explanation for the presenting complaint of fussiness or fever, or (b) substitute shotgun testing for a careful systematic history and physical examination. Both of these approaches are pitfalls in and of themselves as more serious diagnoses can be overlooked or an unnecessary burden of diagnostic testing may be placed on a patient who is typically quite intolerant of anything invasive. In this chapter we review common pitfalls encountered by practitioners evaluating children in the acute care setting and provide clear guidance on how to avoid them.

Pitfall | **Failure to obtain a rectal temperature in the infant**

Fever is defined as a temperature of 38.0 °C (100.4 °F) or greater. Axillary and tympanic temperature measurements in infants and young children are unreliable [1, 2]. Decisions on the appropriate workup of the infant are often based on an accurate temperature measurement. The temperature in the young child should be taken rectally. Bundling of a young infant may increase the skin temperature, but it does not increase the core temperature [3]. The parental assessment of fever by touch is likely to be accurate, but should be confirmed prior to further evaluations.

Pitfall | **Failure to educate parents about the significance of fever**

Parents have many misconceptions and fears about fever, and they should be informed that it is not the height of the fever that is important but how the child looks (toxicity) and any associated symptoms. If a fever doesn't "break" with antipyretics, it does not mean that the infection is more serious. In general, acetaminophen or ibuprofen will bring the fever down 2 or 3 degrees(1–1.5 °C). High fevers (>104 °F, >40 °C) due to infectious causes do not cause brain damage. Body temperatures greater than 108 °F (42.2 °C) can cause brain damage, but those temperatures can only be reached from exogenous heat sources such as being left in an enclosed hot car.

On the other hand, fever in an infant less than 28 days old is very significant and should prompt immediate referral to an Emergency Department. The patient will likely require a complete sepsis evaluation, intravenous antibiotics, and hospital admission. Parents may be concerned about the need for such an invasive evaluation on their child, so it is important to emphasize that neonates have an immature immune system and that fever may be the only sign or symptom of a serious bacterial infection.

For infants of 28 days up to 3 months, many protocols have been developed to identify infants at low

Urgent Care Emergencies: Avoiding the Pitfalls and Improving the Outcomes, First Edition.
Edited by Deepi G. Goyal and Amal Mattu.
© 2012 John Wiley & Sons, Ltd. Published 2012 by John Wiley & Sons, Ltd.

> **Box 11.1** Low-risk criteria for well-appearing febrile infants
>
> *Previously healthy term infants without perinatal complications who are less than 3 months of age and who are not found to have soft tissue, ear, or skeletal infection:*
>
> 1. Nontoxic appearance
> 2. No previous use of antimicrobials
> 3. Lack of a focus of infection on examination
>
> *Low-risk laboratory criteria for well-appearing febrile infants:*
>
> Blood:
>   White Blood Cell (WBC) count between 5,000 and 15,000/mm³
>   Bands less than 1,500/mm³, or
>   Band-to-neutrophil count less than 0.2
>
> Urine:
>   Gram stain negative, or
>   Leukocyte esterase and nitrate negative, or
>   Fewer than 5 WBC/hpf
>
> Cerebral spinal fluid: If performed
>   Gram stain negative
>   Less than 8 WBC/mm³
>
> Chest x-ray: If performed
>   No infiltrate
>
> Stool: If diarrhea present
>   Less than 5 WBC/hpf
>   No blood

Sources: Baker *et al*. [4]; Jaskiewicz and McCarthy [5]; and Baskin *et al*. [6].

risk for serious bacterial infection [4, 5, 6]. The febrile infant less than 2 to 3 months of age who appears "well" may still harbor a serious bacterial illness necessitating a complete sepsis evaluation [4]. If all the studies performed fulfill low-risk criteria (Box 11.1), and parents are reliable for follow-up, the infant may be discharged without antibiotics [4, 7].

In the 1- to 3-month-old febrile infant, the presence of a known viral pathogen such as respiratory syncytial virus (RSV) or influenza significantly decreases the likelihood of concomitant serious bacterial infection. Having a known antigen positive test for RSV reduces the risk for serious

bacterial illness from 9.6 to 2.2% [8]. Similarly, a positive rapid influenza test lowers the risk of serious bacterial infection from 17 to 2.6% [9]. In all cases, the concomitant serious bacterial infection was a urinary tract infection.

This age group may, however, be challenging to manage in an urgent care setting and referrals to and Emergency Department are appropriate.

> KEY FACT | **Well-appearing infants greater than 1 month of age may be discharged to home without antibiotics if they fulfill low-risk history and laboratory criteria, have reliable parents, and have a next day follow-up.**

Pitfall | **Not treating the pain that accompanies an acute ear infection**

Acute otitis media (AOM) is one of the most common infections in childhood. Jointly, the American Academy of Pediatrics and American Academy of Family Practice have set up guidelines for the appropriate diagnosis and management of AOM (Box 11.2). These guidelines stress the importance of accurate diagnosis (certain or uncertain) and subsequent pain management with or without antibiotics. It has been shown that, overall, 60% of children with AOM will have resolution of symptoms in one day, whether treated with antibiotics or placebo [10]. To address the pain associated with AOM, ibuprofen (10 mg/kg every 6 hours) or acetaminophen (15 mg/kg every 4 hours) should be given regularly for the first day after diagnosis. Anesthetic eardrops are also effective at reducing pain. Antipyrine benzocaine combination otic drops, five drops every 3 to 4 hours to the affected ear, has been shown to reduce ear pain compared to placebo [11]. Anesthetic ear drops should not be used if there is any perforation of the tympanic membrane. A diagnosis of *certain* AOM is made if three elements are present: acute onset of symptoms, signs of middle ear effusion, and redness of the tympanic membrane. Severe AOM is defined as having fever (39 °C) or moderate to severe ear pain [12]. Once the decision to start antibiotics is made, the first-line therapy is high-dose amoxicillin

Box 11.2 Criteria to initiate antimicrobial therapy for acute otitis media (AOM)

Treat with Antibiotics at initial presentation:
Six months of age or less whether certain or uncertain AOM
Six months to 2 years of age only if certain diagnosis of AOM

Wait and Watch for 48 to 72 hours:
Uncertain AOM age 6 months to 2 years of age
Certain or uncertain AOM greater than 2 years of age

Treat with Antibiotics at initial presentation if severe pain or fever >39°C:
Uncertain AOM age 6 months to 2 years
Certain AOM greater than 2 years

Certain AOM is defined as acute onset of symptoms, signs of bulging tympanic membrane and inflammation of the tympanic membrane. The wait and watch option consists of treating the pain of the ear infection with topical analgesic ear drops and oral ibuprofen or acetaminophen. A safety net antibiotic prescription (SNAP) may be given at the time of diagnosis and filled at 48 to 72 hours if continued symptoms.

Source: Subcommittee on Management of Acute Otitis Media [12]

(80 mg/kg divided twice daily). Therapy should be for 10 days in children less than 6 years of age, and 5 to 7 days in children 6 years and older. In patients for whom the decision to wait and watch is made, a safety net antibiotic prescription (SNAP) can be given. The SNAP should be filled at 48 to 72 hours only if the child has continued signs and symptoms of ear infection [13]. These symptoms include: persistent ear pain, sleep disruption, crying, fever, or otorrhea. If the child "worsens" during the observation period, the parent should initiate the antibiotics and have the child re-evaluated. Worsening signs and symptoms include; fever >39°C, severe pain, dehydration, lethargy, vomiting, or altered mental status. Regardless of the decision regarding antibiotics, parents should be provided oral and topical analgesics for symptom relief.

KEY FACT | **Over 60% of children with AOM will have resolution of their pain in one day whether treated with antibiotics or placebo.**

Pitfall | Being overly aggressive in obtaining blood cultures on fully immunized, well appearing, febrile child without a source

Vaccination with the conjugated pneumococcal vaccine and the *Haemophilus influenza* type B (HIB) vaccine has dramatically changed the evaluation of the child less than 3 year of age with fever [14]. In 1993, and again in 2003, the American College of Emergency Physicians developed a clinical policy to screen for occult bacteremia to reduce the risk of subsequent serious bacterial illnesses (pneumonia, cellulitis, septic arthritis, osteomyelitis, meningitis, or sepsis) [15, 16]. These guidelines applied to previously healthy, well-appearing children, age 3 to 36 months with fever >39°C without an identifiable source of infection. Since the introduction of the conjugated pneumococcal vaccine in 2000, invasive pneumococcal disease has dramatically declined [17]. Once a child has two conjugated pneumococcal vaccines, which should occur by 4 months of age, the risk for pneumococcal bacteremia is so low that now it is no longer clinically indicated to draw empiric labs and blood culture [7, 18]. The child who is not immunized or has less than two conjugated pneumococcal vaccines is at higher risk of bacteremia, specifically pneumococcal bacteremia. Empiric blood cultures should be considered if the child has a temperature >40°C, petechiae, prolonged gastroenteritis, or contact with meningococcal disease.

KEY FACT | **Well-appearing, febrile children (3 to 36 months), who are fully immunized, with fever (>39°C) without an identifiable source, do not require automatic blood cultures and antibiotics.**

Pitfall | Failure to consider urinary and pulmonary sources of infection in the febrile child

Urinary tract infections (UTIs) – the most common occult infections in children – can present with subtle or no signs or symptoms other than fever. Therefore, consideration of a possible UTI should be given in children presenting with fever >39 °C and no obvious source. Children at highest risk for UTI include: infants <6 months of age, uncircumcised boys <1 year of age, females <2 years of age, and any child with a previous UTI. Factors that increase the sensitivity of detecting a UTI in girls less than 2 years of age are: fever >39 °C, fever for >2 days, white race, and age less than 1 year [19]. Urine should be obtained by urethral catheterization in all children who are not toilet trained. Urine collected by the bag method is unreliable and may be contaminated, leading to unnecessary treatment and testing. Urine testing by dipstick alone may miss a UTI in young children. A Gram stain and urine culture with sensitivities should be performed on all specimens to increase the accuracy of diagnosis and treatment. Antibiotic treatment for UTI depends on local susceptibilities of *E. coli*, the predominant bacteremia in UTIs. Recently, cephalexin has become a first-line oral antibiotic for treatment due to increasing trimethoprim-sulfamethoxazole resistance. Ciprofloxacin is seldom used in children due to the concern for cartilage injury. Infants less than 3 months of age with a urinary tract infection are at high risk for serious bacterial illnesses and should be referred for a possible sepsis evaluation. Infants, 3 months to 1 year with febrile UTI (>39 °C) are also at increased risk of bacteremia and should be considered for referral to an ED for possible blood work and intravenous antibiotics. Referral should also be considered in any child with dehydration or vomiting.

Every child less than 3 years of age with a UTI, should follow-up with their primary care provider for a renal ultrasound and VCUG (voiding cystourethrogram) to detect any congenital renal collecting system abnormalities.

> KEY FACT | **Urine samples in children who are not toilet trained should be obtained by urethral catheterization.**

In children with fever without any obvious source, occult pneumonia is a consideration. Occult pneumonia is defined as a chest x-ray consistent with pneumonia and no respiratory distress or lower airway signs or symptoms. Past fever guidelines recommended obtaining a complete blood count (CBC)

on children less than 3 years of age with fever >39 °C [16]. Children found to have leukocytosis >20,000 per mm³ routinely had a chest x-ray performed. With the implementation of the conjugated pneumococcal vaccine, the incidence of occult pneumonia has decreased from 25% to 5% in highly febrile children with leukocytosis and no signs of pneumonia. Children presenting with only 1 day of fever and no cough are at extremely low risk for occult pneumonia and should not have a chest x-ray performed. The likelihood of detecting pneumonia increases with duration of the cough, worsening cough, duration of the fever and if blood work is obtained, a leukocytosis >20,000 per mm³ [20].

> KEY FACT | **Chest x-rays to evaluate for occult pneumonia should only be considered if the child has had fever for greater than 24 hours.**

Pitfall | **Not assessing the immunization status in children with fever without a source**

Fever greater than 39 °C (102.2 °F) in the unimmunized child is concerning when a focus for the fever cannot be found. If any child appears ill or "toxic," referral should be made to an ED for a full sepsis evaluation and intravenous antibiotics. Even in unimmunized children, the conjugated pneumococcal vaccine has decreased the rate of serious streptococcal infections through herd immunity. None the less, the well-appearing unimmunized child with fever without a source needs to be evaluated for a possible urinary tract infection, occult bacteremia, and pneumonia.

Immunization status does not change the criteria for screening for a urinary tract infection in young children with fever without a source. Catheterized urine should be obtain in females less than 2 years of age, circumcised boys less than 6 months of age, uncircumcised boys less than 1 year of age, and any child with a prior urinary tract infection.

Children less than 3 years of age are at the greatest risk for occult bacteremia. In the unimmunized or under-immunized child, there are two options for further evaluation. One option is to draw a blood culture and administer a dose of ceftriaxone. This approach recognizes that frequently, particularly with meningococcemia and *Salmonella* bacteremia, the WBC count has limited value in predicting illness. The other approach is to obtain a blood culture and CBC with differential: if the WBC count is greater than 15,000 per mm^3, then treat with ceftriaxone [18]; if the WBC count is greater than 20,00 per mm^3, a chest x-ray should be performed to evaluated for occult pneumonia. The child should follow-up the next day for re-evaluation.

> KEY FACT | **A blood culture should be performed in the unimmunized and under-immunized febrile children without a source.**

Pitfall | **Not assessing for oral thrush when an infant has diaper candidiasis**

Infants acquire *Candida albicans* through maternal birth canal exposure, skin contact, and poor bottle sterilization. Over 20% of infants are colonized by the first month of life. Oral thrush in infants produces pain, and consequently poor feeding. On physical examination, oral thrush appears as a white exudate over the inner cheek or tongue. Unlike milk, thrush typically cannot be scraped off with a tongue depressor. *Candida*, once present, colonizes the infant's entire gastrointestinal tract. When breakdown of the skin in the diaper region occurs, infection can take hold. Over 30% of children with candidal diaper dermatitis will have oral thrush simultaneously. Candidal diaper dermatitis starts with redness of the anal mucosa and perianal skin, then spreads over the perineum and in severe cases to the thighs and abdomen. The eruption evolves into scaly papules that coalesce. The distinguishing feature of candidal diaper dermatitis is the presence of *satellite* papules. The satellite lesions are best described as pink to beefy red pustules that spread from the intertriginous area of the diaper toward the legs or abdomen. Treatment for oral thrush is nystatin oral suspension (100,000 units qid) for 1 to 2 weeks. All bottle nipples and pacifiers should be sterilized in boiling water frequently early in therapy. Topical therapy of candidal diaper dermatitis

includes nystatin, miconazole, or clotrimazole. It is important for breast-feeding mothers to apply the antifungal cream to their nipples to decrease reinfection of the infant.

Irritative diaper dermatitis is a very common skin disorder of infancy. Frequently this is due to impairment of the barrier function of the skin: moisture, friction, feces, and microorganisms all play a role. Primary irritative diaper dermatitis usually starts when skin is exposed to moisture for a prolonged period of time. Chemical irritation from urine and feces increases the penetration of bacteria and fungi resulting in severe inflammation. The rash will typically start pink and progress to beefy red as it becomes more severe. Areas of friction and irritation from the diaper are affected most. Typically this will be over the perineum and buttocks, sparing the gluteal cleft and the leg folds. In the areas of greatest irritation, scaling or ulceration may be seen. *Candida albicans* should be considered part of the pathologic process if the irritative dermatitis has been present for greater than 3 days or if the child has recently been on antibiotics [21].

First-line therapies for diaper rash include: increased frequency of diaper changes, superabsorbent disposable diapers, applying water repellant barrier creams (zinc oxide), adding bath oil to bath water, and bathing the baby once or even twice a day. Second-line treatment includes treating with an antifungal ointment such as nystatin, or applying 1% hydrocortisone ointment. Interestingly, the topical antibacterial agent mupirocin applied four times daily works as an antifungal agent and is effective in diaper dermatitis. Other steps include avoidance of irritative diaper wipes that contain fragrance, benzalkonium chloride, and isothiazolinone and alcohol. Warm water, mild soap, and cotton balls are mild and effective for cleaning the diaper area.

> KEY FACT | **The first steps to treat diaper dermatitis are to decrease the moisture in the diaper by frequent changes and to increase the barrier between that moisture and the child with water repellant barrier creams. Children with simultaneous oral and diaper candidiasis should be treated with oral and topical nystatin.**

Pitfall | **Not considering foreign body aspiration in a young child with wheezing**

Foreign body aspiration (FBA) is a potentially life-threatening emergency that has a range of presentations. FBAs are frequently misdiagnosed initially as asthma, pneumonia, choking spell, or upper respiratory infection. The majority of children with FBA will be between the ages of 1 and 3 and will have a sudden onset of coughing or choking. Food items, especially peanuts, are the most common culprits for aspiration. Other common objects aspirated include other nuts and seeds, apples, carrots, and popcorn. On examination the child might have a cough, wheeze, or dyspnea. In young children, the bifurcation mainstem bronchi are at the same angle, making the left bronchus equally open to affection as the right by foreign bodies. Asymmetric breath sounds are heard in the minority of children with FBA. Factors that contribute to delayed diagnosis are lack of a witnessed choking spell and normal radiographs on initial evaluation. Initial radiographs were normal in over 30% of children diagnosed with foreign body aspiration by bronchoscopy. One must maintain a high index of suspicion for FBA in young children, especially in a young child with a choking spell, first time wheezing, or persistent cough. Inspiratory and forced expiratory chest radiographs should be obtained to evaluate for possible air trapping. A normal chest radiograph does not exclude the possibility of a foreign body aspiration; if there is any concern, the child should be referred for further evaluation and possible bronchoscopy.

> KEY FACT | The classic triad of wheeze, cough, and decreased breath sounds is present in only in one-third of cases of pediatric foreign body aspiration.

Pitfall | **Not looking for the double ring sign of a disc battery when a "coin" shaped object is ingested**

Eighty percent of all foreign body ingestions occur in young children (6 months to 3 years of age) due to their curiosity and propensity to explore the world through their mouths [22]. Unlike the older child who is likely to report a history of accidental or intentional foreign body ingestion, young children may have very nonspecific symptoms such as irritability, drooling, food refusal, or may even be asymptomatic. Coins are the most common ingested objects and the vast majority of ingested objects are radiopaque. Management of the ingestion depends not only on the type, size, and shape of the object ingested but also the location of the object upon detection.

Esophageal foreign bodies typically lodge at three distinct points along the esophagus; the level of the cricopharyngeus, thoracic inlet or at the lower esophageal sphincter. Up to 40% of patients with known esophageal coins may be completely asymptomatic. Radiographs of the chest (including a lateral of the chest and neck) and abdomen should be obtained. Esophageal coins will appear as a disc on the AP view and on edge with the lateral view. Care must be taken to differentiate disc batteries from coins as the former can rapidly damage the esophageal mucosa as soon as 1 hour after ingestion. Radiographs of button batteries will have a double density or rim, which is best detected on the lateral view. When identified in the esophagus, immediate removal of a button battery should be performed. Other circular objects lodged in the upper third of the esophagus should be removed within 12–16 hours and sooner if there is airway compromise or distress. Objects in the middle or lower third can be observed for up to 24 hours and will often spontaneously pass. Removal is recommended for impaction greater than 24 hours. An alternative to observation – which can be safely performed in the urgent care setting in selected patients without underlying esophageal abnormalities and known short duration of impaction – is the use of an esophageal dilator (bougienage) to force the object into the stomach. A 95.4% success rate was reported in a retrospective review of 372 patients undergoing bougienage treatment for esophageal coins [23]. This technique was associated with a significant decreased length of stay and cost savings over hospitalization and endoscopy. Sharp objects lodged within the esophagus should be immediately removed typically via rigid or flexible esophagoscopy due to their high risk for perforation and low likelihood of spontaneous passage.

Once an object has entered the stomach, passage is directly related to size and length of the object. Most round objects less than 1 cm by 3 cm will spontaneously pass. Coins in the stomach can be safely observed for 2–4 weeks for spontaneous passage as long as the patient remains asymptomatic. If the object is not identified in the stool within 4 weeks, repeat radiographs to confirm passage or retention are recommended. Endoscopic removal of a coin that has not passed out of the stomach by this time is generally recommended. Long, non-sharp objects may pass even if they are up to 5–6 cm in length as long as their diameter is less than 2 cm. Sharp objects in the stomach or proximal duodenum are often removed due to the higher risk of perforation (up to 35%) but once these objects have moved beyond the duodenal sweep, observation is recommended unless signs of perforation such as fever or peritoneal signs develop. Consultation with a gastroenterologist for any identified or suspected ingested sharp object in the stomach, no matter what the size, is reasonable.

Magnets used in children's toys have become more common and present a unique problem when ingested. While a single smooth edged magnet poses little to no risk, multiple magnets can attach to each other across loops of bowel, creating an obstruction. Radiographic evidence of more than one magnet in the stomach, unless these magnets are already attached to each other, should prompt immediate removal. Once magnets have traversed the pylorus, careful observation for signs of bowel obstruction, or development of significant abdominal pain that could indicate perforation, would guide surgical removal.

> KEY FACT | **90% of all ingested foreign bodies will pass spontaneously. Only 1% will require surgical intervention.**

Pitfall | **Failure to use a systematic approach to the evaluation of the fussy, well appearing infant**

There are few diagnostic dilemmas more challenging than the well-appearing fussy or crying infant.

Box 11.3 Some potential causes of fussiness in a well appearing infant

HEENT
Corneal abrasion; oral candidiasis; coxsackie viral herpangina; herpes gingivostomatitis; otitis media

Gastrointestinal/Genitourinary
Constipation; intussusception; gastroesophageal reflux; rectal fissure; hernia; testicular torsion; urinary tract infection

Cutaneous
Hair tourniquet; skin or soft tissue abscess; diaper dermatitis: group A streptococcal perianal dermatitis, candida, contact dermatitis

Miscellaneous/Other
Recent immunizations; abuse; supraventricular tachycardia; infantile colic

---

Parents of these children often want answers as to why their child is crying excessively and may themselves be quite emotional. A provider can quickly become overwhelmed by these emotions, or the fear of missing a potentially devastating diagnosis, and embark on a rabbit trail of testing. Alternatively, there may be a tendency to prematurely label the child as having infantile colic before ruling out other possibilities. Colic is a diagnosis of exclusion, thus it is important to rule out a variety of other causes for the crying infant. An astute clinician armed with a good differential and a thorough physical examination can rule in or out most of the common causes for the well-appearing crying infant. Additional testing can be based on the presence or absence of other findings (Box 11.3).

Corneal abrasions are common yet quite difficult to detect without fluorescein staining. An infant will not necessarily present with unilateral tearing but may have asymmetric redness of one eye and the crying is typically sudden in onset. Crying will often resolve after instillation of an ophthalmic anesthetic prior to placement of the fluorescein which confirms the diagnosis. Oral candidiasis can be a normal finding in infants and is sometimes asymptomatic. When associated with poor feeding, a trial of antifungals can be initiated. Coxsackie viral infection (herpangina) or primary herpes gingivostomatitis may have subtle initial presentations, so close examination of the oral cavity should not be overlooked. Otitis media is often overcalled as a cause of crying in an infant. The diagnosis should be certain, based on clinical findings including pneumatic otoscopy. Treatment of the pain with numbing ear drops and oral analgesics should produce resolution of the crying if otitis is indeed the cause.

Intermittent fussiness in a somewhat predictable or rhythmic pattern can be seen in infants with constipation. A careful history of stooling frequency and consistency along with a digital rectal examination will provide important clues in making this diagnosis. Close examination of the rectal mucosa for a rectal fissure is done at the same time. Intussusception can also produce similar symptoms as constipation. Infants may be completely normal in between episodes and a high index of suspicion is required. Intussusception, however, is relatively rare under 6 months of age. When suspected, plain radiographs and sometimes a confirmatory ultrasound or diagnostic air or contrast enema are necessary to diagnose this condition.

Timing of the onset of crying can provide important clues. Infants that become very fussy shortly after eating with associated arching of the back and turning of their head (Sandifer syndrome) may suffer from gastroesophageal reflux. There usually is a clear association with feedings. A trial of acid-blocking agents can help to confirm this diagnosis. Certain routine immunizations are also associated with fussiness. Diphtheria–tetanus–acellular pertussis (DTaP), conjugated pneumococcal, and oral rotavirus vaccines all indicate fussiness or irritability as common side effects on the vaccine information sheets. DTaP has also been associated with nonstop crying for greater than 3 hours in 1 out of 1,000 infants administered this vaccine.

It is critically important to completely undress the infant to search for hair or other fiber tourniquets, which can be found on any of the digits, penis, labia, or even clitoral regions. A thorough skin examination looking for bruising may indicate the possibility of abuse. Intraoral bruising or tearing of the frenulum are very concerning findings in infants for abuse. A complete musculoskeletal examination may highlight an area of swelling or tenderness associated with a fracture or redness and swelling secondary to a septic joint. Attention to the diaper region is also important, looking for subcutaneous abscesses seen in community acquired methicillin-resistant *Staphilococcus aureus*. This organism has a predilection for the diaper region in infants due to rectal colonization. Severe diaper dermatitis caused by group A beta hemolytic streptococcus, candida species, or even contact dermatitis can be painful and produce crying. Genitourinary examination looking for scrotal or labial swelling, if nonreducible, may indicate an incarcerated or strangulated inguinal hernia. An abnormal testicular lie with swelling suggests testicular torsion.

Supraventricular tachycardia in infants is often asymptomatic. However, if an infant is found to have an extreme tachycardia with no identifiable cause to suggest a compensatory sinus tachycardia, an ECG looking for the absence of p-waves, and a rhythm strip to identify the absence of variability, should be obtained. Signs of heart failure are late phenomena in the otherwise healthy infant with no underlying structural heart abnormalities.

When no source for the crying can be identified, in the infant under 3 months of age a urinary tract infection should be ruled out with a catheterized specimen, even in the absence of fever. Other routine laboratory or imaging testing is not recommended.

> KEY FACT | **Thorough examination, not extensive testing of the fussy or crying infant, is essential in localizing a source for the discomfort.**

Pitfall | **Over utilization of neuroimaging of the minor head-injured child**

Traumatic brain injury is one of the leading causes of death and disability in children world wide. In the United States alone there are an estimated 1.5–3.8 million head injuries in children each year. The vast majority of these injuries are minor yet there still remains a small but significant percentage

Table 11.1 Decision rule for identifying children at low risk for clinically important traumatic brain injury (ciTbI)

Age < 2 years		
GCS = 14 or other signs of altered mental status* or signs of depressed skull fracture	→	CT scan indicated (4.4% risk of ciTBI)
Nonfrontal scalp hematoma, or history of LOC ≥ 5 s, or severe mechanism of injury,** or not acting normally per parent	→	Consider observation vs CT scan (0.9% risk of ciTBI)
None of the above risk factors	→	CT scan not indicated (< 0.02% risk of ciTBI)
Age 2 years to 18 years		
GCS = 14 or other signs of altered mental status* or signs of basilar skull fracture	→	CT scan indicated (4.3% risk of ciTBI)
History of LOC, or history of vomiting, or severe mechanism of injury,** or severe headache	→	Consider observation vs CT scan (0.9% risk of ciTBI)
None of the above risk factors	→	CT scan not indicated (< 0.05% risk of ciTBI)

*Agitation, somnolence, repetitive questioning, or slow to respond to verbal communication.
**Motor vehicle crash with patient ejection, death of another passenger, or rollover; pedestrian or bicyclist without a helmet struck by a motorized vehicle; falls of more than 3 (age < 2) or 5 ft (age > 2); or head struck by high impact object.
Modified from Kuppermann *et al.* [24] with permission from Elsevier.

of patients with relatively unimpressive presenting signs or symptoms that have suffered a clinically important injury. Equally important is the increased awareness of the radiation risks associated with excessive CT usage.

Identification of the child that is at low risk for clinically important traumatic brain injury (ciTBI) is necessary for the acute care provider, both to identify important injuries and to minimize over-testing or referral. There is a great deal of parental and provider anxiety over missing these injuries which has contributed to a dramatic rise in the use of CT scanning. Concurrently, there has also been a recognition and growing concern over the potential risks of ionizing radiation to the developing brain. Recently, a robust clinical decision rule with a negative predictive value for ciTBI of 100% was prospectively derived and validated and published to assist providers in the evaluation of this patient population (Table 11.1) [24]. The authors identified higher risk factors and lower risk factors for ciTBI and, based on these findings,

nicely described a tiered approach to patients. For example, a child over 2 years of age with only vomiting would not necessarily require neuroim-aging as the risk for ciTBI is less than 0.9%. In this case, the authors recommend a period of observation versus imaging, based on clinician experience. Utilization of this prediction rule could dramatically decrease the exposure of children to potentially harmful ionizing radiation or unnecessary referral for imaging.

Pitfall | **Failure to manage concussions according to guidelines**

A concussion is defined as a complex pathophysiological process affecting the brain, induced by traumatic biomechanical forces [25]. Clinically more important are some key features of concussions that assist in making the diagnosis. A concussion can be sustained either through a direct blow to the head or neck or through transmitted impulsive forces such as from a blow to the body or from rapid deceleration in a motor vehicle accident. Loss of consciousness is not a prerequisite to a diagnosis that is clinically based on the presence of symptoms in one or more of the following realms: physical, cognitive, emotional, or sleep related. Lists of commonly reported symptoms within these categories are widely available, and symptoms of concussion typically fall into one of those four realms. While patients can complain of a host of different types of physical symptoms, the most commonly reported ones are headache, nausea, vomiting, imbalance, visual problems, fatigue, sensitivity to light or sounds, and feeling "stunned." Cognitive symptoms may manifest as feeling mentally "foggy", sluggish or slow; concentration difficulties; confusion, forgetfulness, or repetitive questioning; and slowness while answering questions. Patients with concussion will often report the presence of emotional lability, sadness, nervousness, or even a flattened affect. Excessive sleepiness or drowsiness, difficulty falling asleep or staying asleep, are some of the sleep-related disturbances associated with concussions [25].

It is important to note that neurological dysfunction represents a functional and not a structural disturbance, and thus most patients with a concussion will have completely normal neuroimaging if obtained. Thus, a negative CT scan, or falling into the low-risk category based on a clinical decision, does not rule out the possibility of a patient still having a concussion.

When a patient meets the clinical diagnosis of a concussion, it is not necessary to attempt to assign a "grade" to the concussion [25]. The currently accepted approach to determining the timing of return to activity is based on the evaluation of symptom resolution rather than concussion grading. Thus, the clinician must be able to identify patients who have sustained a concussion and appropriately refer them for follow-up. For the more severely affected patients it may be necessary to impose both physical and cognitive restrictions to minimize symptoms and speed recovery. The magnitude of these restrictions (i.e. complete versus partial physical and cognitive rest) should be recommended by the initial provider, but the duration of these restrictions are tailored to the individual and cannot be accurately predicted ahead of time. Close follow-up is essential. Most concussive symptoms are short lived, with the vast majority of patients experiencing complete resolution in 7–10 days. Patients with repeated concussions or delayed presentation to care, and a history of a mechanism consistent with a probable concussion and prolonged symptoms, may require immediate referral to a specialist in dealing with traumatic brain injury. All other cases can be referred back to the primary care provider.

KEY FACT | Utilizing a simple clinical decision rule for minor head injury can significantly reduce the use of CT scans in children presenting with minor head injury but does not rule out the possibility of a concussion.

Pearls for improving patient outcomes

• The clinical appearance of a young infant (<2–3 months) presenting with fever is not reliable in determining whether a sepsis evaluation should be performed to evaluate for serious bacterial illnesses.

• Parents should be given weight-based dosing of ibuprofen or acetaminophen to treat pain or fever effectively.

• The majority of ear infections are viral in nature and only require adequate pain control with ibuprofen or acetaminophen and otic drops, not antibiotics.

• Fully immunized, well-appearing children (<36 months) with high fever (>39 °C) for more than 2 days and no apparent source of infection on history or physical examination, should have a urine and or a chest x-ray performed to evaluate for a possible occult bacterial infection.

• Diaper rash is the result of skin breakdown due to an overly moist diaper environment. To effectively treat it, a strong barrier cream, superabsorbent diapers and frequent diaper changes should be used.

• Foreign body aspiration should be considered in any young children with a history of choking spell or sudden onset coughing illness. Radiographs are frequently "normal." If the suspicion is high, referral should be made for bronchoscopy.

• With any coin lodged in the esophagus, always consider the possibility that it may be a disc battery. Look for the distinctive double ring that is seen with batteries.

• Colic is a diagnosis of exclusion; fussy infants require a thorough stepwise evaluation.

• Utilization of a simple clinical decision rule can help to classify patients with minor closed head injury into low risk, very low risk, and high risk groups to guide imaging decisions.

• Concussion is a clinical diagnosis. Patients diagnosed with a concussion should have limitations in their physical and cognitive activity and should be fully recovered prior to return to sport activities.

References

1 Yetman RJ, Coody DK, West MS, *et al.* Comparison of temperature measurements by an aural infrared thermometer with measurements by traditional rectal and axillary techniques. *J Pediatr* 1993; **122**(5): 769–773.

2 Muma BK, Treloar DJ, Wurmlinger K, *et al.* Comparison of rectal, axillary, and tympanic membrane temperatures in infants and young children. *Ann Emerg Med* 1991; **20**(1): 41–44.

3 Grover G, Berkowitz CD. The effects of bundling on infant temperature. *Pediatrics* 1994 11; **94**(5): 669.

4 Baker MD, Bell LM, Avner JR. The efficacy of routine outpatient management without antibiotics of fever in selected infants. *Pediatrics* Mar 1, 1999; **103**(3): 627–631.

5 Jaskiewicz JA, McCarthy CA. Febrile infants at low risk for serious bacterial infection – an appraisal of the Rochester. *Pediatrics* 1994 Sep; **94**(3): 390.

6 Baskin M, O'Rourke E, Fleisher G. Outpatient treatment of febrile infants 28 to 89 days of age with intramuscular administration of ceftriaxone. *J Pediatr* 1992; **120**(1): 22–27.

7 Baraff L. Management of infants and young children with fever without source. *Pediatr Ann* 2008 Oct; **37**(10): 673–679.

8 Bilavsky E, Shouval D, Yarden-Bilavsky H, *et al.* A prospective study of the risk for serious bacterial infections in hospitalized febrile infants with or without bronchiolitis. *Pediatr Infec Dis J* 2008; **27**(3): 269–270.

9 Mintegi S, Garcia-Garcia J, Benito J, *et al.* Rapid influenza test in young febrile infants for the identification of low-risk patients. *Pediatr Infec Dis J* 2009; **28**(11): 1026–1028.

10 Rosenfeld R, Kay D. Natural history of untreated otitis media. *Laryngoscope* 2003; **113**(10): 1645–1657.

11 Hoberman A, Paradise JL, Reynolds EA, Urkin J. Efficacy of auralgan for treating ear pain in children with acute otitis media. *Arch Pediatr Adolesc Med* 1997 July 1; **151**(7): 675–678.

12 Subcommittee on Management of Acute Otitis Media. Diagnosis and management of acute otitis media. *Pediatrics* 2004 May 1, 2004; **113**(5): 1451–1465.

13 Johnson NC, Holger JS. Pediatric Acute otitis media: the case for delayed antibiotic treatment. *J Emerg Med* 2007; **32**(3): 279–284.

14 Joffe M, Alpern E. Occult pneumococcal bacteremia – a review. *Pediatr Emerg Care* 2010; **26**(6): 448–454.

15 Baraff LJ, Bass JW, Fleisher GR, *et al.* Practice guideline for the management of infants and children 0 to 36 months of age with fever without source. *Ann Emerg Med* 1993; **22**(7): 1198–1210.

16 Clinical policy for children younger than three years presenting to the emergency department with fever. *Ann Emerg Med* 2003; **42**(4): 530–545.

17 Wilkinson M, Bulloch B, Smith M. Prevalence of occult bacteremia in children aged 3 to 36 months presenting to the emergency department with fever in the postpneumococcal conjugate vaccine era. *Acad Emerg Med* 2009; **16**(3): 220–225.

18 Ishimine P. The evolving approach to the young child who has fever and no obvious source. *Emerg Med Clin North Am* 2007; **25**(4): 1087–1115.

19 Gorelick M, Hoberman A, Kearney D, *et al.* Validation of a decision rule identifying febrile young girls at high risk for urinary tract infection. *Pediatr Emerg Care* 2003; **19**(3): 162–164.

20 Shah S, Mathews B, Neuman M, Bachur R. Detection of Occult Pneumonia in a Pediatric Emergency Department. *Pediatr Emerg Care* 2010; **26**(9): 615–621.

21 Gökalp A, Aldirmaz C, Oğuz A, *et al.* Relation between the intestinal flora and diaper dermatitis in infancy. *Trop Geogr Med* 1990; **42**(3): 238–240.

22 Wyllie R. Foreign bodies in the gastrointestinal tract. *Curr Opin Pediatr* 2006; **18**: 563–564.

23 Arms J, Mackenberg-Mohn M, Bowen M, *et al.* Safety and efficacy of a protocol using bougienage or endoscopy for the management of coins acutely lodged in the esophagus: a large case series. *Ann Emerg Med* 2008; **51**(4): 367–372.

24 Kuppermann N, Holmes J, Dayan P, *et al.* Identification of children at very low risk of clinically-important brain injuries after head trauma: a prospective cohort study. *Lancet* 2009; **374**(9696): 1160–1170.

25 Halstead M, Walter K, The Council on Sports Medicine and Fitness. Sport-related concussion in children and adolescents. *Pediatrics* 2010; **126**(3): 597–615.

CHAPTER 12
Geriatric Pitfalls

Joseph P. Martinez
Department of Emergency Medicine, University of Maryland School of Medicine, Baltimore, MD, USA

Introduction

The world's population is aging rapidly. By the year 2025, it is estimated that there will be 1.2 billion people in the world over the age of 60. The "oldest old" (people over the age of 80) is the fastest growing subgroup of the population. By 2050, the oldest old will account for 4% of the world's population, up from the current 1% [1]. Despite these numbers, it is clear that urgent and emergent care of the elderly remains suboptimal. In the European heat wave of 2003 where nearly 30,000 people died, France had 14,800 deaths with 75% of those deaths occurring in people over 75 years old [2]. In Hurricane Katrina, 71% of the deaths in Louisiana were in people over the age of 60 [3].

Elderly patients pose unique challenges to acute care practitioners. Common diseases often present atypically in the elderly, laboratory values are frequently unhelpful, comorbid conditions may complicate even relatively straightforward medical issues, and social support systems may make it difficult for patients to handle even seemingly innocuous problems such as sprained ankles.

Pitfall | **Failure to appreciate atypical presentations of acute coronary syndrome**

> KEY FACT | **The most common "atypical" symptoms of ACS in the elderly are dyspnea, diaphoresis, nausea/vomiting, and syncope. Only 35% of patients over the age of 84 will have an ST-elevation myocardial infarction as their presentation of ACS.**

It is well-documented that acute coronary syndrome (ACS) can present atypically in the elderly. People over the age of 60 account for 65% of all cases of ACS and 80% of all deaths. In the Global Registry of Acute Coronary Events (GRACE registry), 8.4% of patients with ACS presented without chest pain. Those patients without chest pain were significantly older than those presenting with chest pain. Of the subset of patients without chest pain, nearly one-quarter were not initially recognized as having ACS. The most common presenting symptoms in those patients without chest pain were dyspnea, diaphoresis, nausea and vomiting, and syncope (see Table 12.1) [4]. The mortality rate of patients presenting atypically was 13% as opposed to 4.3% in the typical group (p<0.001). Elderly patients also have a higher incidence of "silent ischemia." This has been shown in autopsy studies where significant coronary artery stenosis is seen in 50% of patients over the age of 80, although only 20% had demonstrated clinical disease while living

Urgent Care Emergencies: Avoiding the Pitfalls and Improving the Outcomes, First Edition.
Edited by Deepi G. Goyal and Amal Mattu.
© 2012 John Wiley & Sons, Ltd. Published 2012 by John Wiley & Sons, Ltd.

[5]. In addition, the elderly have longer intervals from time of symptom onset and are more likely to have nondiagnostic electrocardiograms [6]. While younger patients have ST-elevation myocardial infarctions (STEMIs) as their presentation of ACS about 80% of the time, the elderly more commonly have non-STEMIs. Only 35% of those above the age of 84 will have a STEMI as their presentation of ACS [7] (Figure 12.1).

Table 12.1 Most common symptoms that manifest as atypical presentations of ACS

Symptom	Percentage of time symptom is seen in cases of "atypical" ACS
Dyspnea	50%
Diaphoresis	26%
Nausea/vomiting	24%
Syncope	19%

(Note, some cases of ACS present with more than one symptom, so percentages do not total 100)

Costochondritis is a condition where the costochondral or chondrosternal junctions become inflamed causing anterior chest pain and tenderness on palpation. A benign condition, it is usually treated with analgesics, reassurance, and rest. It is common practice for practitioners to palpate the chest wall of patients presenting with chest pain, especially if they are otherwise well appearing. Tenderness on palpation often prompts the practitioner to label the pain "musculoskeletal" or "costochondritis." However, 6–8% of acute myocardial infarctions will have chest wall tenderness on examination [8]. In a study where patients were considered to have "noncardiac chest pain" after history, physical examination, and electrocardiogram, nearly 3% went on to have a definite adverse cardiac event with another 3.5% having a possible adverse cardiac event [9]. The patients that were mislabeled were an average of 13 years older, with a mean age of 61.1 years. It is with extreme caution (if ever) that a geriatric patient should be labeled as having "costochondritis" without further evaluation for more serious pathology.

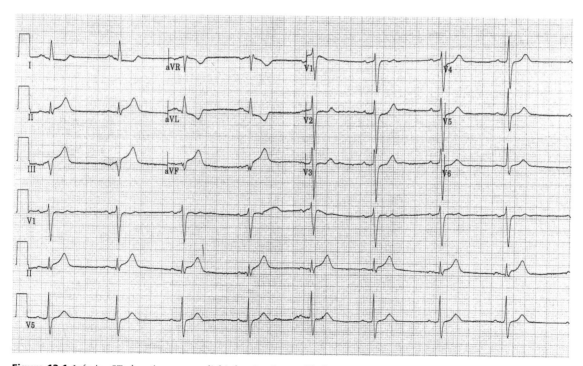

Figure 12.1 Inferior ST-elevation myocardial infarction in an elderly patient that presented with nausea and vomiting but absence of chest pain. The elderly often present without pain during acute coronary syndrome.

Pitfall | **Misinterpretation of "normal" vital signs**

Most practitioners evaluate a patient's vital signs as the first step of any encounter. However, this seemingly straightforward practice may be fraught with hazards in the case of the geriatric patient. "Normal" vital signs may lead to delays in triage, evaluation, and resuscitation of geriatric patients. It is hard to define what "normal" is in this patient population, and when values are abnormal, it may be difficult to assess how significant this is. Elderly patients are often normothermic or even hypothermic despite serious infectious pathology [10]. Tachycardia that would normally be expected with some serious conditions may be absent due to intrinsic conduction system abnormalities or may be blunted by medications such as beta-blockers. Recent literature has highlighted the importance of tachycardia in geriatric trauma patients where even mild tachycardia was associated with dramatic increases in the mortality rate of the elderly population [11]. Chronic hypertension is one of the most common diseases afflicting mankind, with a prevalence of up to 80% in people over the age of 70 [12]. A "normal" blood pressure may represent significant hypoperfusion in a patient with underlying hypertension. There has been a great deal of evidence in the trauma literature showing that occult hypoperfusion in geriatric patients can be seen with systolic blood pressures in the range of 130–150 mmHg [13]. A recent study of nearly 25,000 patients from the Los Angeles County Trauma Database identified the optimal definition of hypotension after trauma as being 120 mmHg in patients aged 50 to 69 years and 140 mmHg in patients 70 years and older [14]. Pain is often described as the "fifth vital sign." Even in this, the elderly may not be as reliable. Altered pain perception among this population is well documented. A study from the 1960s demonstrated a prolongation in time necessary to both sense a painful stimulus and then to perceive it as painful [15]. Endoscopically proven peptic ulcer disease is painless only 8% of the time in young cohorts, but in patients above the age of 60 it may be seen in up to 35% of cases [16].

Pitfall | **Minimizing geriatric abdominal pain**

Elderly patients with abdominal pain are among the most high-risk patients that an acute care provider will encounter. In some studies, the mortality rate of an elderly patient presenting with abdominal pain is higher than that of the same patient presenting with chest pain. Yet, too often, providers make the costly error of trivializing this complaint or attributing symptoms to a lesser illness such as gastroenteritis. The reasons for this are myriad. The elderly patient often presents very atypically which leads to frequent misdiagnoses. It may be more difficult to take an adequate history in elderly patients due to dementia, hearing loss, or stoicism. Elderly patients often take more medications than younger patients. These medications may mask pathology or be the cause of pathology. As was discussed earlier, vital signs may be less reliable in the elderly. So too, is the physical examination. The abdominal musculature is thin in elderly patients. This leads to a decrease in rigidity and guarding, even in cases of frank peritonitis. Laboratory values may falsely reassure the less seasoned provider. Nearly one-quarter of cases of appendicitis in the elderly and 40% of cases of acute cholecystitis will have normal white blood cell counts [17, 18]. Laboratory values may also be misleading: red blood cells seen on urinalysis may represent nephrolithiasis, but they can also be seen in cases of ruptured abdominal aortic aneurysms.

Peptic ulcer disease

As previously noted, the elderly can have endoscopically proven peptic ulcer disease without symptoms. One-half of all ulcers in the elderly will have a complication (e.g. a perforation or acute bleed) as their presenting symptom [19]. Perforations present very differently in the elderly than in younger patients. Acute onset of pain is found in only one-half of cases. The rigid, board-like abdomen that many expect to find is actually noted in a small minority of cases of perforated ulcers, roughly 20% [20]. Free intraperitoneal air on plain radiographs is seen in less than one-half of cases [21] (see Figure 12.2). Elderly patients

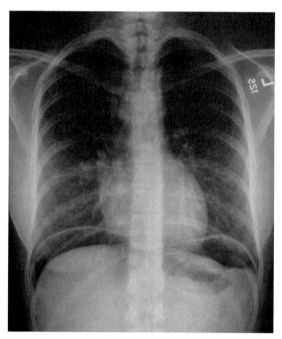

Figure 12.2 Free intraperitoneal air in a patient with a perforated gastric ulcer. Of note, only 40% of elderly with a perforated viscus will have free air on plain radiographs.

fare worse than younger patients with conservative treatment [22]. They are more likely to bleed from their ulcers, to require blood transfusions, and to require surgery to control the bleeding [23]. All of these factors lead to a mortality rate from peptic ulcer disease three times as high in the geriatric population as compared to younger patients [24].

> KEY FACT | **Less than one-quarter of cases of perforated viscus will present with frank rigidity.**

Biliary tract disease

The most common reason for acute abdominal surgery in the elderly, biliary tract disease can also be challenging to diagnose. While most geriatric patients will present with tenderness in the right upper quadrant or epigastrium, other supporting evidence may be absent. More than half of elderly patients with acute cholecystitis will not have

nausea or vomiting and half will be afebrile [18]. White blood cell counts and liver function tests are frequently normal. While ultrasound remains a reasonable screening test, the elderly are at higher risk for acalculous cholecystitis, which is not as easily appreciated on ultrasound. Thus, consideration of a radionuclide (HIDA) scan should be made in any elderly patient with a suspicion of acute cholecystitis and a negative ultrasound.

Choledocholithiasis is also more common in the elderly and with it, ascending cholangitis. Acute suppurative cholangitis is rarely seen before the seventh decade. This diagnosis mandates emergent decompression, either through surgery, endoscopy, or percutaneous drainage. Disseminated intravascular coagulation is common in these disorders.

Appendicitis

Thought by many to be a disease of the young, acute appendicitis is the third most common indication for abdominal surgery in the elderly [25]. Despite its lower incidence in this population, the elderly account for 50% of all deaths from appendicitis [26]. Acute appendicitis is notoriously difficult to diagnose in the elderly. Elderly patients tend to present later with one-fifth presenting after 3 days of symptoms and another 5–10% after one week of symptoms [27]. Only 20% of geriatric patients will present with classic findings of fever, right lower quadrant pain, and leukocytosis. Fever is absent in two-thirds, right lower quadrant tenderness is absent in 30%, and leukocytosis is absent in one-quarter [28]. Fully one-quarter of all cases of appendicitis in the elderly are misdiagnosed at first provider contact and inappropriately discharged home [28]. It is not surprising then that mortality rates are 4–8% in this population (compared to 1% in younger patients) and perforation rates are a staggering 70%! [29]. Liberal use of CT scanning is encouraged in this age group if the patient still possesses an appendix (see Figure 12.3).

> KEY FACT | **One-quarter of all cases of acute appendicitis in the elderly are missed at first presentation to an acute care provider.**

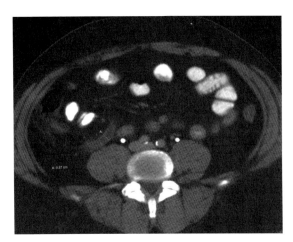

Figure 12.3 Dilated appendix that is not filling with oral contrast, consistent with acute appendicitis.

Mesenteric ischemia

Mesenteric ischemia is a life-threatening disorder resulting in hypoperfusion of the gut. It can be caused by an embolus lodged in the superior mesenteric artery (SMA), a thrombosis that forms in the SMA, a venous thrombosis, or a low-flow state (nonocclusive mesenteric ischemia). The majority of cases are due to an SMA embolus. They present acutely with abdominal pain, which is classically out of proportion to the physical examination. "Gut emptying" is frequently seen in cases of mesenteric ischemia. This refers to vomiting, diarrhea, or both and may explain why the most common misdiagnosis of mesenteric ischemia is gastroenteritis. Although atrial fibrillation is the classic source of emboli, in reality, it is seen on less than 50% of cases [30]. An important diagnostic clue on history is that one-third of patients with an SMA embolus will have had a prior embolic event. Thrombosis of the SMA typically occurs in patients with atherosclerosis risk factors. Plaque builds at the origin of the SMA where there is turbulent flow. Patients may relate a history of "intestinal angina," which is post-prandial abdominal pain. This may cause "food fear" where patients avoid eating and lose significant amounts of weight. Similar to acute coronary syndrome, plaque rupture leads to the acute onset of abdominal pain akin to an SMA embolus. Eliciting the history of intestinal angina or "food fear" may help to make the diagnosis. Mesenteric venous thrombosis will often present less acutely with symptoms lasting days to weeks before diagnosis. These patients may have an underlying hypercoaguable state and one-half will have a personal or a family history of venous thromboembolic disease. Nonocclusive mesenteric ischemia is seen in low-flow states such as sepsis, dehydration, or severe cardiomyopathy. It may also be seen in hemodialysis patients or patients using digitalis [31].

> KEY FACT | **One-half of patients with mesenteric venous thrombosis will have a personal or a family history of venous thromboembolic disease.**

The diagnosis of mesenteric ischemia is enormously challenging. Physical examination is usually unhelpful early in the course. Do not be falsely reassured by a soft abdomen in patients with a concerning history or risk factors for this disease. Mislabeling them as gastroenteritis will likely lead to death as the mortality from mesenteric ischemia remains near 80%. Patients suspected of having mesenteric ischemia should be sent for emergent angiography and surgical consultation. Similar to ACS, time is of the essence in these cases. Angiography before the onset of peritoneal signs can dramatically decrease the mortality rate [32, 33]. As multidetector row CT angiography continues to evolve, it will likely become a good screening test for patients at low or moderate risk (see Box 12.1).

Ruptured abdominal aortic aneurysm

Ruptured abdominal aortic aneurysm (AAA) is another great imitator in the geriatric population. While the diagnosis may be fairly straightforward in the patient with hypotension, abdominal pain, and pulsatile abdominal mass, this presentation occurs in a small minority of cases. Hypotension is absent in 65% of cases [34]. The pain may be confined to the back or flank instead of the abdomen, and

---

Box 12.1 Types of mesenteric ischemia and historical clues

SMA embolus
One-third of cases have had a previous embolic event

SMA thrombosis
Typical atherosclerosis risk factors
History of intestinal angina or "food fear"

Mesenteric venous thrombosis
Presents less acutely
One in two have a personal or family history of venous thromboembolism

Nonocclusive mesenteric ischemia
Low-flow sates
Often ICU patients
Association with digitalis use and hemodialysis

SMA = superior mesenteric artery

---

palpable pulsatile masses are often absent or missed on physical examination. The most common misdiagnosis is renal colic. This is easy to understand in a patient that presents with flank pain radiating toward the groin and microscopic hematuria (caused by irritation of the ureter by the enlarging AAA). Other frequent misdiagnoses include musculoskeletal back pain and diverticulitis. The misdiagnosis rate is as high as 30–50% [35, 36]. Elderly patients presenting with new-onset "renal colic" should undergo imaging of their aorta, either with ultrasound or computed tomography.

KEY FACT | **Hypotension is absent in 65% of cases [of ruptured AAA].**

Pitfall | **Underappreciating the morbidity and mortality associated with "simple" falls**

The most common reason for trauma in the elderly is falls [37]. The leading cause of death from injury in patients over the age of 65 is complications from falls. The overall mortality from falls is about 11% [38]. Low-level falls (standing height) account for the majority of falls. As can be seen from this data,

even "low-impact" falls in the elderly are high-risk events than can lead to serious morbidity and mortality.

The bones of elderly patients are less able to withstand mechanical forces of trauma. Mechanisms of injury thought to be "low-impact," such as falls from standing position, can result in significant injuries to the geriatric patient. Coexisting osteoporosis may lead to an increased risk of fracture. Decrease in skin functions leads to increased injury and decreased protection from infection. The aging brain decreases in both size and weight. This results in stretching of bridging vessels on the surface of the brain, which can then tear from relatively minor shearing forces. Patients may be taking blood thinners or antiplatelet agents that increase their risk of bleeding. All of the above mandates that the acute care provider take falls seriously and perform a thorough evaluation for serious injury.

The cause of the fall must also be investigated. While many falls are mechanical due to environmental causes such as steps, area rugs, and thresholds, unexplained falls must be treated as syncope. In patients with syncope from cardiovascular causes, 20% will present merely with unexplained falls [39]. Falls from underlying illnesses including serious entities such as myocardial infarction or vascular catastrophes should also be considered. Alcohol disorders are found in 10–15% of elderly patients presenting to emergency departments and may contribute to falls [40]. Acute care providers must always be vigilant for the possibility of elder abuse as a cause of "falls."

CNS injuries

There are no validated guidelines for evaluating elderly patients with blunt head injury. As noted above, the elderly are at much greater risk for intracranial pathology due to the physiologic changes in brain and bone that accompany aging. The presentation of traumatic injury in geriatric patients may be occult. Of 1,934 patients above the age of 65 in the National Emergency X-Radiography Utilization Study (NEXUS) II trial [41], 178 (9.2%) had significant intracranial injury. Forty-four percent of

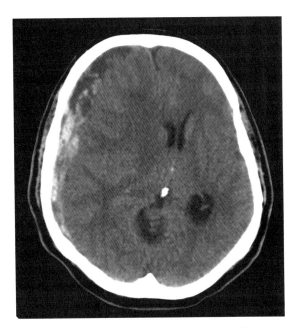

Figure 12.4 Right subdural hematoma with midline shift in an elderly patient on warfarin who presented after a fall from standing.

these patients had no focal neurologic deficits. A small (2.2%) but significant proportion of patients had occult injury, defined as normal level of consciousness, no neurologic deficit and no evidence of skull fracture. This presentation was seen in only 0.8% of younger patients [41]. The investigators were "unable to identify criteria that could reliably be used to detect or exclude injury in elders." The incidence of injury was even higher in patients on anticoagulation. The liberal use of CT imaging is advised in this patient population (see Figure 12.4).

Fractures

Fractures complicate 5–10% of all falls in the elderly [42]. Forearm fractures are the most common fractures in women while hip fractures are the most common in men and overall [43]. Vertebral fractures, pelvic fractures, and rib fractures are also seen more commonly in this age group. The presence of hip pain or the inability to ambulate despite negative plain radiographs should

prompt consideration of occult hip fracture. Nearly 5% of patients with these complaints and negative plain radiographs will have an occult fracture found on advanced imaging [44]. Patients unable to ambulate after a fall should not be discharged without further evaluation or observation.

Low-level falls lead to increased risk of injury to the spine in the levels between occiput and C2 [45]. A recent study found that clinical predictors were inadequate for evaluating geriatric patients with low-level injuries [46]. Indeed, the Canadian C-Spine rule considers all patients above the age of 65 to be high-risk and recommends routine radiographic evaluation in this group [47]. The presence of a cervical spine fracture is associated with increased morbidity and mortality (up to 25%), regardless of whether there is associated spinal cord injury or other traumatic injuries [48]. The mortality from elderly patients with rib fractures is twice that of younger patients. Even a single rib fracture has significant morbidity and mortality associated. With each successive rib fractured, mortality and the risk of pneumonia increase. If elderly patients have 3 rib fractures, their mortality is roughly 20% and risk of pneumonia is 31%. If they have 6 rib fractures, their mortality climbs to 33% and over half of them will develop pneumonia [49]. Truly, these are high-risk injuries.

> KEY FACT | **Rib fractures are associated with significant morbidity and mortality in the elderly, and these rates increase with each successive rib fractured.**

Pitfall | **Failing to consider elder abuse**

While elder abuse is usually recognized in the most obvious cases, the great majority of cases are more subtle and often the abuse goes unrecognized. First described in the medical community in 1975, elder abuse has finally become recognized as a distinct entity and is now the subject of much research [50, 51]. Abuse may take many forms: physical, sexual, or psychological as well as neglect, abandonment, exploitation and violation of personal rights. Abuse can occur in the elderly person's domicile or in an institutional setting. Actual numbers are hard to quantify due to reporting problems, but it is estimated that at least 3–5% of all elders have been victimized at some point, with the most common type of abuse being neglect [52–54]. By far, the most likely perpetrator is a close relative, with adult children committing abuse in nearly one-half of all cases and a spouse being the abuser in one-fifth [55]. Alcoholism or other substance abuse by the perpetrator is the most predictive characteristic [56, 57].

Most acute care practitioners do not routinely ask elderly patients about abuse or neglect, though it has been shown that this simple act can increase detection. Careful physical examination may uncover clues such as bruises in various stages of healing (especially if not over bony prominences), burns, patterned injuries such as hand slaps or ligature marks, or signs of neglect including infestation or untreated injuries. Radiographs may be warranted and may show signs of acute or remote fractures. A low threshold for neuroimaging should be maintained in cases of suspected abuse as significant injuries can occur from shaking or low-level falls.

Various areas have different reporting requirements, and it is imperative to be familiar with the regulations where you practice. Regardless of local requirements, it is a moral imperative for any acute care provider not to discharge a patient back to a setting that they feel is unsafe for the patient.

Conclusion

The elderly are at high risk for presenting with atypical symptoms. Vital signs may appear normal and physical examination may be unremarkable, despite serious illness. Since patients may be non-toxic in appearance, it is common to attribute their symptoms to a benign cause. This is a practice that should be discarded in the elderly population, who often are hiding serious pathology. There are certain diagnoses that the astute practitioner should be particularly cautious with in the elderly population. Costochondritis and gastroenteritis are diagnoses that should give the acute care clinician particular pause when used in the elderly. Falls are

very common in this population. Even low-impact falls such as from a standing or sitting position can lead to serious injuries. Every acute care provider that cares for geriatric patients should be vigilant for possible elder abuse.

Pearls for improving patient outcomes

• An electrocardiogram should be obtained early in the care of any elderly patient presenting with vague complaints including unexplained dyspnea, nausea/vomiting, or diaphoresis.
• Be aggressive when confronted with abnormal vital signs and do not attribute them simply to pain.
• Consider mesenteric ischemia any time you plan to diagnose an elderly patient with "gastroenteritis." Reconsider this diagnosis if they have risk factors for mesenteric ischemia or complaints of severe pain (which is not typically seen in gastroenteritis).
• Any elderly patient being diagnosed with a first episode of nephrolithiasis should have their aortic size assessed, either with computed tomography or ultrasound.
• Every geriatric patient that presents with an injury should be screened for elder abuse.

References

1 Wells J. Protecting and assisting older people in emergencies. *Humanitarian Practice Network*. London: Overseas Development Institute, 2005.
2 International Red Cross and Red Crescent Societies. *World Disaster Report 2004: Focus on Community Resiliency*. Bloomfield: Kumarian Press, 2004.
3 American Association of Retired Persons (AARP). *We Can Do Better: Lessons Learned from Protecting Older Persons in Disasters*. Washington: AARP Public Policy Institute, 2006.
4 Brieger D, Eagle K, Goodman S, *et al.* Acute coronary syndromes without chest pain, an underdiagnosed and undertreated high-risk group. *Chest* 2004; **126**: 461–469.
5 Elveback L, Lie JT. Continued high incidence of coronary artery disease at autopsy in Olmsted County, Minnesota, 1950 to 1979. *Circulation* 1984; **70**: 345–349.
6 Kyriades ZS, Kourouklis S, Kontaras K. Acute coronary syndromes in the elderly. *Drugs Aging* 2007; **24**(11): 901–912.

7 Cheitlin MD, Zipes DP. Part VII, Chapter 57: Cardiovascular disease in the elderly. In: *Braunwald's Heart Disease: A Textbook of Cardiovascular Medicine* (6th edn.). Philadelphia (PA): Saunders Company, 2001: 2019–2037.

8 Disla E, Rhim HR, Reddy A, *et al.* Costochondritis. A prospective analysis in an emergency department setting. *Arch Intern Med.* 1994; **154**(21): 2466–2469.

9 Miller CD, Lindsell CJ, Khandelwal S, *et al.* Is the initial diagnostic impression of "noncardiac chest pain" adequate to exclude cardiac disease? [Published correction appears in *Ann Emerg Med* 2005; **45**(1): 87]. Ann Emerg Med 2004; **44**(6): 565–574.

10 Fenyo G. Diagnostic problems of acute abdominal diseases in the aged. *Acta Chir Scand* 1974; **140**: 396–405.

11 Heffernan DS, Thakkar RK, Monaghan SF, *et al.* Normal presenting vital signs are unreliable in geriatric blunt trauma victims. *J Trauma* 2010; **69**: 813–820.

12 Chobanian AV, Bakris GL, Black HR, *et al.* Seventh Report of the Joint National Committee on Prevention, Detection, Evaluation, and Treatment of High Blood Pressure. *Hypertension* 2003; **42**: 1206–1252.

13 Scalea T, Simon H, Duncan A, *et al.* Geriatric blunt multiple trauma: improved survival with early invasive monitoring. *J Trauma* 1990; **30**: 129–134.

14 Edwards M, Let E, Mirocha J, *et al.* Defining hypotension in moderate to severely injured trauma patients: raising the bar for the elderly. *American Surgeon* 2010; **76**: 1035–1038.

15 Sherman ED, Robillard E. Sensitivity to pain in the aged. *Can Med Assoc J* 1960; **83**: 944–947.

16 Leverat M. Peptic ulcer disease in patients over 60: experience in 287 cases. *Am J Dig Dis* 1966; **11**: 279–285.

17 Horattas MC, Guyton DP, Wu D. A reappraisal of appendicitis in the elderly. *Am J Surg* 1990; **160**: 291–293.

18 Morrow DJ, Thompson J, Wilson SE. Acute cholecystitis in the elderly. *Arch Surg* 1978; **113**: 1149–1152.

19 Caesar R. Dangerous complaints: the acute geriatric abdomen. *Emerg Med Rep* 1994; **15**: 191–202.

20 Fenyo G. Acute abdominal disease in the elderly: experience from two series in Stockholm. *Am J Surg* 1982; **143**: 751–754.

21 McNamara RM. Acute abdominal pain. In: Sanders AB (ed.), *Emergency Care of the Elder Person.* St. Louis: Beverly Cracom Publications; 1996: pp. 219–243.

22 Crofts TJ, Park KG, Steele RJ. A randomized trial of nonoperative treatment for perforated peptic ulcer. *N Engl J Med* 1989; **320**(15): 970–973.

23 Borum ML. Peptic-ulcer disease in the elderly. *Clin Geriatr Med* 1999; **15**: 457–471.

24 Wakayama T. Risk factors influencing the short-term results of gastroduodenal perforation. *Surg Today* 1994; **24**(8): 681–687.

25 Kauvar DR. The geriatric acute abdomen. *Clin Geriatr Med* 1993; **9**: 547–545.

26 Shoji BT, Becker JM. Colorectal disease in the elderly patient. *Surg Clin N Am* 1994; **74**: 293–316.

27 Freund HR, Rubinstein E. Appendicitis in the aged: is it really different? *Am Surg* 1984; **50**: 573–576.

28 Storm-Dickerson TL, Horratas MC. What have we learned over the past 20 years about appendicitis in the elderly? *Am J Surg* 2003; **185**: 198–201.

29 Yamini D, Vargas H, Bongard F, *et al.* Perforated appendicitis: is it truly a surgical urgency? *Am Surg* 1998; **64**: 970–975.

30 Park WM, Gloviczki P, Cherry KJ Jr, *et al.* Contemporary management of acute mesenteric ischemia: factors associated with survival. *J Vasc Surg* 2002; **35**(3): 445–452.

31 Diamond S, Emmett M, Henrich WL. Bowel infarction as a cause of death in dialysis patients. *JAMA* 1986; **256**: 2545–2547.

32 Boley SJ, Sprayregen S, Siegelman SJ, Veith FJ. Initial results from an aggressive roentgenologic and surgical approach to acute mesenteric ischemia. *Surgery* 1977; **82**: 848–855.

33 Clark RA, Gallant TE. Acute mesenteric ischemia: angiographic spectrum. *AJR Am J Roentgenol* 1984; **142**: 555–562.

34 Rutherford RB, McCroskey BL. Ruptured abdominal aneurysm: special considerations. *Surg Clin North Am* 1989; **69**: 859–868.

35 Marston WA, Ahlquist R, Johnson G Jr, *et al.* Misdiagnosis of ruptured abdominal aortic aneurysms. *J Vasc Surg* 1992; **16**: 17–22.

36 Salkin MS. Abdominal aortic aneurysm: avoiding failure to diagnose. *ED Legal Letter* 1997; **8**: 67–78.

37 Aschkenasy MT, Rothenhaus TC. Trauma and falls in the elderly. *Emerg Med Clin North Am* 2006; **24**: 413–432.

38 Mosenthal AC, Livingston DH, Elcavage J, *et al.* Falls: epidemiology and strategies for prevention. *J Trauma* 1995; **38**: 752–756.

39 Mitchell LE, Richardson DA, Davies AJ, *et al.* Prevalence of hypotensive disorders in older patients with a pacemaker in situ who attend the accident and emergency department because of falls or syncope. *Europace* 2002; **4**: 143–147.

40 O'Connell H, Chin AV, Cunningham C, *et al.* Alcohol use disorders in elderly people – redefining an age old problem in old age. *BMJ* 2003; **327**: 664–667.

41 Rathlev NK, Medzon R, Lowery D, *et al*. Intracranial pathology in elders with blunthead trauma. *Acad Emerg Med* 2006; **13**: 302–307.

42 van Weel C, Vermeulen H, van den Bosch W. Falls, a community care perspective. *Lancet* 1995; **345**: 1549–1551.

43 Nordell E, Jarnlo G, Jetsen C, *et al*. Accidental falls and related fractures; A retrospective study of 332 patients. *Acta Orthop Scand* 2000; **71**(2): 175–179.

44 Dominguez S, Liu P, Roberts C, *et al*. Prevalence of traumatic hip and pelvic fractures in patients with suspected hip fracture and negative initial standard radiographs - a study of emergency department patients. *Acad Emerg Med* 2005; **12**(4): 366–369.

45 Sharma OP, Oswanski MF, Yazdi JS, Jindal S, Taylor M. Assessment for additional spinal trauma in patients with cervical spine injury. *Am Surg* 2007; **73**(1): 70–74.

46 Schrag SP, Toedter LJ, McQuay N. Cervical spine fractures in geriatric blunt trauma patients with low-energy mechanism: are clinical predictors adequate? *Am J Surg* 2008; **195**: 170–173.

47 Stiell IG, Wells GA, Vandemheen KL, *et al*. The Canadian C-Spine rule for radiography in alert and stable trauma patients. *JAMA* 2001; **286**: 1841–1848.

48 Golob JF, Claridge JA, Yowler CJ, *et al*. Isolated cervical spine fractures in the elderly: a deadly injury. *J Trauma* 2008; **64**: 311–315.

49 Bulger EM, Arneson MA, Mock CN, Jurkovich GJ. Rib fractures in the elderly. *J Trauma* 2000; **48**: 1040–1046.

50 Burston GR. Granny-battering. *BMJ* 1975; **3**: 592.

51 Baker AA. Granny battering. *Mod Geriatr* 1975; **5**: 20–24.

52 Pillemer K, Finkelhor D. The prevalence of elder abuse: a random sample survey. *Gerontologist* 1988; **29**: 51–57.

53 Davidson JL. Elder abuse. In: Block MR, Sinnott JD (eds.), *The Battered Elder Syndrome: An Exploratory Study*. College Park (MD): University of Maryland; 1979: pp. 49–66.

54 Lachs MS, Williams C, O'Brien S, *et al*. Risk factors for reported elder abuse and neglect: a nine-year observational cohort study. *Gerontologist* 1997; **37**: 469–474.

55 United States Department of Health and Human Services Administration on Aging and the Administration for Children and Families. *The National Elder Abuse Incidence Study*. Washington (DC): NCEA, 1998.

56 Kosberg JI, Nahmiash D. Characteristics of victims and perpetrators and milieus of abuse and neglect. In: Baumhover LA, Beall SC (eds.), *Abuse, Neglect, and Exploitation of Older Persons: Strategies for Assessment and Intervention*. Baltimore (MD): Health Professions Press; 1996: pp. 31–49.

57 Lachs MS, Pillemer K. Abuse and neglect of elderly persons. *N Engl J Med* 1995; **332**: 437–443.

CHAPTER 13

Pharmacology Pitfalls and Pearls in Urgent Care Medicine

Christopher E. Anderson and Ronna L. Campbell
Department of Emergency Medicine, Mayo Clinic, Rochester, MN, USA

Introduction

The U.S. Food and Drug Administration Adverse Events Reporting System reported over 60,000 deaths in 2009 due to medication adverse events or errors, making medication-related problems the eighth leading cause of death in the U.S. [1, 2]. Adverse drug events account for 17 million emergency department visits in the United States annually. Costs associated with adverse drug events totaled $177 billion in 2000. A recent study revealed that 12% of visits to a tertiary emergency department were drug-related, and 68% of these events were preventable. Preventable adverse drug events involve incorrect dosing; a known allergy; a known interaction; nonadherence; lack of laboratory monitoring; and prescribing, dispensing, or administrative errors [3]. Furthermore, several medications can have side effects that cause unneeded anxiety among patients and providers. Knowledge of these common adverse effects can prevent anxiety by providing patients with proper anticipatory guidance. Finally, certain populations need special consideration to mitigate medication pitfalls.

Pitfalls and pearls in pharmacology of commonly used medications

Analgesics
Nonsteroidal anti-inflammatory drugs

Pitfall | **Failure to recognize patients at risk for gastrointestinal and renal complications from NSAIDs**

Nonsteroidal anti-inflammatory drugs (NSAIDs) work by inhibiting one or both cycloxygenase (COX) enzymes. COX enzyme inhibition results in both the untoward and therapeutic NSAID effects. In the kidney, COX-1 produces prostacyclins that maintain renal blood flow. In the gastrointestinal tract, COX-1 produces a prostacyclin that enhances mucosal perfusion, bicarbonate production and mucous production, which contribute to mucosal integrity. NSAIDs are the second most common cause of peptic ulcer formation behind *Helicobacter pylori* infection [4–6] (see Box 13.1).

Urgent Care Emergencies: Avoiding the Pitfalls and Improving the Outcomes, First Edition.
Edited by Deepi G. Goyal and Amal Mattu.
© 2012 John Wiley & Sons, Ltd. Published 2012 by John Wiley & Sons, Ltd.

> **Box 13.1** Contributing factors to NSAID-induced kidney and GI injury [5, 6]
>
> *Conditions that predispose to NSAID-induced kidney injury*
>
> Dehydration
>
> Reduced urine output
>
> Impaired renal function
>
> ACE inhibitors
>
> ARBs
>
> Diuretics
>
> *Conditions that predispose to NSAID-induced GI injury*
>
> History of GI bleed
>
> Peptic ulcer disease
>
> Age > 60
>
> High doses of NSAID
>
> Glucocorticoids
>
> Anticoagulants

Acetaminophen

Pitfall | Failure to recognize atypical products that contain acetaminophen

More than 200 medication combinations contain acetaminophen as a component. Typical recommendations for maximal daily dosage are 3 g/day in adults and 75 mg/kg/day in children. A small amount of acetaminophen is normally metabolized by the liver into a highly hepatotoxic metabolite. Normally, protective mechanisms rapidly metabolize these toxic products. With excessive acetaminophen ingestion, these can be overwhelmed resulting in hepatotoxicity. Usually a 7.5 g or 150 mg/kg or greater dose is required to cause hepatotoxicity. Patients with liver dysfunction or those with chronic supratherapeutic ingestions are at greater risk for toxicity. Chronic overdose or usual doses in patients with liver dysfunction can cause toxicity. Many chronic ingestions can be inadvertent as many combination preparations contain acetaminophen. Opioid-acetaminophen combinations as well as over-the-counter combinations with NSAIDs, sedatives, and other agents (e.g. Midrin ®, Excedrin ®, etc.) exist. If acute acet-

aminophen toxicity is suspected, a serum level should be obtained 4 hours after the time of ingestion (in cases of acute ingestion) and plotted on the Rumack–Matthew nomogram to determine if n-acetylcysteine antidote therapy is required [7]. The Rumack–Matthew nomogram does not apply to chronic overdose. A patient should be treated for acetaminophen toxicity if chronic overdose is suspected and liver function tests are abnormal [8]. Consultation with a toxicologist or poison control center is strongly recommended if patients with suspected toxicity are not transferred to a higher level of care.

> KEY FACT | **Over-the-counter analgesics can cause significant toxicity, some of which can present occultly.**

Opioids

Pitfall | Failure to adequately manage pain

Although, pain is the most common reason people seek emergency care, many patients do not receive adequate analgesia in acute care settings. There are many reasons why providers fail to manage pain. Among these are failure to acknowledge and assess pain, failure to use pain management guidelines, failure to assess treatment adequacy, and concerns about addiction or dependence [9]. In a recent multicenter study, 40% of patients in significant pain received no analgesia. When analgesia was given, it occurred on average 90 minutes after the patient was at triage. Because patients often do not voice their desire for analgesics, each patient should be asked about pain severity and whether they want analgesics [10].

Studies have documented racial and gender disparities in analgesia administration in emergency departments. At one center, nonwhites were more likely to report severe pain yet less likely to receive analgesia. White patients were 10% more likely to receive opiates and had a shorter wait for opiates than nonwhites [11]. Likewise, women were less likely to receive analgesia, had greater delays to

Table 13.1 Opioid analgesic dosing

Agent	Dose equivalent to morphine 10 mg IM		Recommended initial dose*
	Parenteral	Oral	
Morphine sulfate	10 mg	60 mg	0.1 mg/kg IV every 1–2 h
Hydrocodone	15 mg	30 mg	5–10 mg PO every 4–6 h
Hydromorphone	1.5 mg	8 mg	0.5 mg IV every 2–3 h
Oxycodone	15 mg	30 mg	5–15 mg PO every 4–6 h
Fentanyl	0.1 mg	NA	1 mcg/kg IV every 30–60 min

*Appropriate opioid dosing can vary widely. The lowest adequate dose should be used. Patient factors such as tolerance, comorbidities (e.g. renal function, hepatic function) and concurrent adjunctive therapies should be taken into account when dosing opioids. Data from Lowell [4], Micromedex® Healthcare Series [7], and Tietze [16]

analgesia, and were less likely to receive opiates than were men with similar pain scores [12]. Providers should strive to appropriately and adequately manage pain. Patients should be asked to rate their level of pain, and treatment should be tailored to meet their needs.

Opioids are the most effective analgesics for certain types of pain. They have an essential role in the urgent care setting. However, opioid analgesics do possess less desirable properties such as tolerance, addiction, and withdrawal. Nonmedical opioid use has paralleled the increase in opioid prescribing [13]. Drug-seeking behavior often poses a challenge for urgent care practitioners. In each case, the risk of inappropriate use of a narcotic must be weighed against the risk of under-treating a patient's legitimate pain. Although studies have not identified predictors of aberrant drug-related behavior, opioids are rarely misused when administered under proper supervision [14]. Inappropriate opioid use was found in only 3.8% of patients receiving opioids for degenerative arthritis, low back pain, migraine, neuropathy, or fibromyalgia. A study examining long-term use of controlled-release oxycodone in patients with chronic pain found only a 2.6% misuse rate [15]. When the legitimate need for opioid analgesia is uncertain, it may be appropriate to provide a short course of opiates and recommend rapid primary care follow-up. (See Table 13.1 [4,7,16].)

Local anesthetics

Pitfall | Failure to recognize the potential catastrophic effects of overdose and intravascular injection

Overdose or intravascular injection of local anesthetics can cause severe side effects including seizures and arrhythmias. Central nervous system (CNS) intoxication is characterized by muscle twitching followed by generalized tonic–clonic seizure activity. In massive overdose, apnea and coma are seen. Arrhythmias and contractile dysfunction are manifestations of local anesthetic cardiovascular toxicity. A centrally mediated mechanism may also produce bradycardia and hypotension [17].

Awareness of the maximum safe dose for a local anesthetic will prevent toxicity. Special attention should be paid when using local anesthetic for large injuries or when repeat dosing is needed. Intravascular injection can quickly lead to toxic levels. Aspiration of the needle prior to injection is 98% effective at identifying intravascular placement [18]. Local anesthetics can be combined with epinephrine to improve hemostasis, increase duration of action, and increase the toxic threshold [19].

Pitfall | Failure to differentiate classes of local anesthetics when an allergy to a local anesthetic exists

Table 13.2 Local anesthetics

	Maximum dose	Notes
Amides		
Lidocaine	4.5 mg/kg; 7 mg/kg with epinephrine	1% lidocaine contains 10 mg/mL
Bupivacaine	2 mg/kg; 3 mg/kg with epinephrine	–
Mepivacaine	4 mg/kg	Only supplied with epinephrine
Prilocaine and lidocaine cream (EMLA)	–	For use on intact skin. Apply under a semi-occlusive dressing.
Lidocaine (4%), epinephrine (0.1%), and tetracaine (0.5%) (LET)	–	For use on open skin.
Esters		
Procaine	7 mg/kg; 9 mg/kg with epinephrine	–
Chloroprocaine	8 mg/kg	–
Cocaine	150 mg for a 70 kg adult	Used only in the nose, nasopharynx, mouth, throat, and ear
Benzocaine spray (20% solution)	–	Potential to cause methemoglobinemia
Proparacaine	1 drop at a time until adequate anesthesia is obtained	For ophthalmologic use

Data from [19, 20]

There are two chemical classes of local anesthetics: amides and esters (Table 13.2). Patients with allergies to an agent are typically allergic to all agents of the same group, but may safely be given an anesthetic of the other group [4]. In the rare case that allergy exists to both amides and esters, diphenhydramine 1% can be used as an alternative local anesthetic for wound repair [20,21].

Pitfall | **Failure to ameliorate pain of injection of local anesthetics**

Local anesthetics have low pH and cause pain on injection. Numerous studies have evaluated the effects of buffering, warming, and rate of injection on pain created by the injection itself [22–24]. Addition of 8.4% sodium bicarbonate can reduce time to onset and decrease pain with injection by raising pH. The dose of sodium bicarbonate should not exceed 1 mL per 9 mL of 1% lidocaine and 1 mL per 20 mL of 0.25% bupivacaine [21]. Warming and a slower rate of injection also decreases pain on injection. Attempts should be made to use all three strategies when administering local anesthetics.

KEY FACT | **Attention to pain management is an important aspect of emergency care. Care must be taken to use them most effectively and safely.**

Antiemetics

Ondansetron

Pitfall | **Administering ondansetron to patients with QT prolongation**

Prescribers should be familiar with the potential for drug-induced ventricular arrhythmias. Certain medications are known to prolong the electrocardiogram (ECG) QT interval, which is a risk factor for developing tachyarrhythmias. Medications from several classes – including antiemetics, antiarrhythmics, antibacterials, and antipsychotics – carry a risk of drug-induced ventricular arrhythmias [25]. One example of a QT-prolonging medication is ondansetron, which works centrally and peripherally to decrease nausea. It lacks many of the side effects

Box 13.2 QTc prolonging medicines

High risk of prolonging QTc

Amiodarone	Methadone
Droperidol	Quinidine
Erythromycin	Sotalol

Possibly prolong QTc

Dronedarone	Ondansetron
Escitalopram	Quetiapine
Fosphenytoin	Risperidone
Levofloxacin	Tacrolimus
Lithium	Tamoxifen
Nicardipine	Vardenafil
	Venlafaxine
	Ziprasidone

(e.g. akathesia) associated with other antiemetics [26] and is available in IV, PO (tablet and liquid), and oral-dissolving preparations. Ondansetron should be avoided in patients with a prolonged QT interval as it has been shown to increase the QT interval by approximately 17 ms and has been associated with the induction of fatal ventricular tachycardia [27–30]. The following are steps to prevent ventricular arrhythmia secondary to QT prolongation:

1 If a patient's baseline ECG demonstrates QTc prolongation (>450 ms in men and 470 ms in females), avoid QTc-prolonging agents.

2 If a patient does not have a baseline ECG available, be mindful of items in the patient's history that might suggest QTc prolongation. These include a history of syncope or arrhythmia, ischemic heart disease, cardiomyopathy, or congestive heart failure. If a QTc-prolonging agent is being considered, obtain a screening ECG prior to administration.

3 If a patient is taking or is starting a medication that is known to prolong the QT interval, consider using another agent or obtaining an ECG to ensure that the patient does not have baseline QT prolongation. Common medications that prolong the QT interval are listed in Box 13.2. Avoid combinations of drugs that are known to prolong the QT interval. The Arizona Center for Education and Research on Therapeutics publishes updated lists of drugs that can

potentially cause drug-induced torsades de pointes. The list can be accessed at: http://www.azcert.org/medical-pros/drug-lists/bycategory.cfm# [31].

4 If a QTc-prolonging drug is already being used, avoid medications that cause hypokalemia or hypomagnesemia, or agents that inhibit the drug's metabolism [30].

Prochlorperazine

Pitfall | **Failure to recognize and treat prochlorperazine-induced akathesia**

Prochlorperazine exerts its effect by blocking dopaminergic receptors, which can also result in extrapyramidal side effects such as akathesia [26, 32]. Akathesia is a syndrome characterized by a subjective feeling of inner restlessness and an inability to remain still. The symptoms of akathesia are variable, ranging from a mild sense of anxiety to severe discomfort. Akathesia can be subtle and mistaken for impatience. Patients may become restless and leave due to the effects of akathesia. Akathesia is induced in up to 40% of patients receiving a 10 mg dose of IV prochlorperazine [33]. Studies have shown that the risk of akathesia can be reduced by administration of diphenhydramine [34]. Patients should be warned about the possibility of akathesia and be frequently monitored. If the patient describes a sensation of anxiety or restlessness after receiving prochlorperazine, he or she should be treated appropriately with diphenhydramine. In a study of emergency department patients, a 50-mg dose of IV diphenhydramine virtually eliminated akathesia in patients receiving parenteral prochlorperazine. One must be mindful of the adverse effects of diphenhydramine, including anticholinergic effects, cognitive decline, and sedation [33].

> KEY FACT | **Antiemetics must be used carefully to avoid potentially catastrophic effects.**

Antibiotics

Pitfall | **Failure to consider the risks and benefits of prescribing antibiotics**

Many patients with upper respiratory tract infections expect to be prescribed an antibiotic, and this expectation has been shown to increase antibiotic prescriptions [35]. However, educational campaigns aimed at providers and patients have successfully decreased antibiotic prescribing. Furthermore, it has been shown that withholding antibiotics does not decrease patient satisfaction [36, 37].

Upper respiratory tract infections (acute otitis media, purulent rhinitis, pharyngitis, common cold, and acute sinusitis) can have viral, bacterial, or mixed etiology and are generally self-limited diseases. In group A streptococcal pharyngitis, antibiotics reduce the incidence of acute rheumatic fever by two-thirds, however, total symptom duration is only shortened by 16 hours. Treatment of only proven (or highly suspected based on diagnostic criteria) group A streptococcal pharyngitis is important to avoid antibiotic resistance. Evidence for efficacy of antibiotics for acute sinusitis is mixed. Guidelines recommend antibiotics only for patients with moderate to severe symptoms and symptomatic treatment and reassurance for those with mild disease [38]. In acute otitis media, antibiotics reduce pain but have no impact on hearing and rarely shorten the course of disease. As these conditions are typically self-limited, a "wait-and-see" strategy for antibiotics may be appropriate for populations with poor access to healthcare or who have not improved with conservative therapy. This strategy significantly reduces antibiotic use compared to immediate prescribing. Benefits of withholding antibiotics include decreased diarrhea, vomiting, rash, and antibiotic resistance [39].

The widespread use of antibiotics has led to unpleasant and sometimes lethal side effects. For instance, the antibiotic-associated intestinal infections caused by *Clostridium difficile* range from diarrhea to life-threatening colitis. Infection with this toxin-producing organism is becoming progressively more frequent, more severe, more refractory to standard therapy, and more likely to relapse. *Clostridium difficile* (*C. diff*)is now the most common bacterial cause of diarrhea. Risk factors include antibiotic exposure, advanced age, and hospitalization. Clindamycin, ampicillin, cephalosporins, and, more recently, fluoroquinolones are most frequently implicated, but almost any antibiotic can induce disease. Common presenting complaints include diarrhea, abdominal cramps, and fever. Fecal leukocytes are seen and leukocytosis is usually present. Disease severity can range from diarrhea to fulminant pseudomembranous colitis, which can lead to toxic megacolon, shock, and potentially death. Antibiotic restraint is essential to minimize the risk of this potentially deadly disease [40].

Another undesirable consequence of antibiotic overuse is the accelerated emergence of bacterial resistance. New strains of bacteria resistant to multiple classes of antibiotics (i.e. "superbugs") are steadily increasing. In the past, the problem of resistance was primarily confined to hospitals and nursing homes. However, more recently, resistant bacteria have been recognized as a significant cause of community-acquired infections. Methicillin-resistant *Staphylococcus aureus* (MRSA) is an increasingly important cause of skin and soft tissue infections and pneumonia. A recent study of emergency department patients found that nearly half of patients with community-acquired skin or soft tissue infection were infected or colonized with MRSA. Fortunately, most strains of community-acquired MRSA are susceptible to trimethoprim-sulfamethoxazole, doxycycline, or clindamycin [41]. The prevalence of other antibiotic-resistant community-acquired infections is also increasing. Examples include pneumonia, urinary tract infections, and sexually transmitted diseases, among others.

Cephalosporins

Pitfall | **Failure to recognize potential cross-reactivity between cephalosporins and penicillins**

Cephalosporins share a beta-lactam ring that is present in penicillins [42]. Patients who have had anaphylaxis, Stevens–Johnson syndrome, toxic epidermal necrolysis, angioedema, or other potentially life-threatening reactions to a penicillin should not receive a cephalosporin. Package inserts for cephalosporins state that cross-hypersensitivity occurs in up to 10% of patients with penicillin allergy, but more recent studies that suggest that this may be an overestimate of the problem [40, 43]. It is generally safe to prescribe a cephalosporin to a patient with a non-life-threatening reaction to penicillin. Nevertheless, routine use of cephalosporins in patients with a penicillin allergy is discouraged by professional societies unless the patient has had a negative penicillin skin test [44]. The higher the generation of cephalosporin the lower the likelihood of penicillin cross-reactivity [45].

> KEY FACT | **Antibiotics can have significant adverse effects and should only be used when indicated.**

Important adverse reactions

Pitfall | Failure to consider fall risk when prescribing medications with psychotropic effects

Diazepam and other benzodiazepines are frequently prescribed for a number of indications including muscle spasm, anxiety, alcohol withdrawal, and insomnia. The sedative effect has a propensity to increase the risk of falls, particularly in the elderly [46]. Thirty percent of people older than 65 years fall at least once per year and the result can be devastating. Long-acting benzodiazepines have been associated with increased risk of hip fractures and hypnotics as a class have been found to be associated with falls [47, 48].

Psychotropic medications have also been associated with increased falls. Selective serotonin reuptake inhibitors (SSRIs) are more strongly related to falls than tricyclic antidepressants. The mechanism may be related to the sedative effect or orthostatic hypotension. Antipsychotics have also been associated with falls, possibly due to sedation, extrapyramidal gait disturbance, or anticholinergic visual disturbance. Interestingly, most studies have concluded that antihypertensives do not increase fall risk. Although, codeine has been linked to an increased risk of hip fracture, no association between opioids (semisynthetic opiate derivatives such as oxycodone, hydromorphone, and hydrocodone) and falls has been reported [47].

Hypnotics, antidepressants, and benzodiazepines demonstrate a significant association with falls in the elderly. Thus, alternatives should be used whenever possible.

Pitfall | Failure to consider a drug reaction in patients presenting with rash

Classic medication reaction patterns include: drug induced exanthems, urticaria (IgE-mediated), serum sickness, vasculitis, Stevens–Johnson syndrome (SJS), photosensitivity and others.

The typical drug-induced exanthema is usually morbilliform (measles-like exanthema with discrete maculopapules) or macular papular. It often begins in dependent areas and then generalizes. It is commonly pruritic and usually occurs within 2 weeks of taking a new drug or within days of re-exposure.

Stevens–Johnson syndrome (SJS), also known as erythema multiforme major, and toxic epidermal necrolysis (TEN) are potentially fatal conditions that cause the epidermis to separate from the dermis. Although most cases are idiopathic, the most common known cause is medications. Medications that are known to precipitate SJS include antigout agents (especially allopurinol), antibiotics (sulfonamides, penicillins, cephalosporins, and others), antipsychotics, antiepileptics (including carbamazepine, phenytoin, lamotrigine, phenobarbital), analgesics including nonsteroidal anti-inflammatory agents, and certain antineoplastic drugs. SJS has a mortality rate of approximately 5%. SJS must be strongly considered in any patient presenting with new erythematous skin lesions who is taking a medication known to precipitate SJS. In these cases, the suspected medication should be stopped until SJS is ruled out [49].

Warfarin

Pitfall | Failure to consider warfarin interactions when prescribing medications.

Warfarin is a commonly used vitamin K antagonist. It is metabolized by the p450 pathway in the liver. Because this pathway metabolizes many medications, many medications affect warfarin's metabolism. Some medications increase its metabolism, potentially leading to life-threatening thromboembolic disease. Others inhibit its metabolism, potentially leading to life-threatening bleeding

Box 13.3 Commonly prescribed medications that interact with warfarin

Increased effect

Acetaminophen	Fluconazole
Allopurinol	Fluoxetine (and other SSRIs)
Aspirin	Glucagon
Amiodarone	Influenza virus vaccine
Cephalosporins	Metronidazole
Cimetidine	Macrolide antibiotics
Ciprofloxacin	Omeprazole
Clopidogrel	Sulfamethoxazole-
Diclofenac	trimethoprim
Erythromycin	Thyroid hormone

Decreased effect

Carbamazepine	Nafcillin
Dicloxacillin	Oral contraceptives
Haloperidol	Phenobarbital
	Vitamin K

[50]. Warfarin is in the top two medications implicated in adverse drug events. Nearly 30,000 patients taking warfarin present to emergency departments each year for bleeding [51].

Several antibiotics increase the effect of warfarin (see Box 13.3). Caution must be used when prescribing fluoroquinolones, trimethoprim/sulfamethoxazole, metronidazole, fluconazole, and azithromycin [52–55]. Increased anticoagulation is typically seen within the first week of therapy. The American Geriatrics Society recommends more frequent monitoring once any antibiotic is started [56]. There are no studies on the specific timing of monitoring; however, consider recommending that patients have an INR checked within 4 days of starting any antibiotic, and perhaps sooner in high-risk patients (initiation of high-risk antibiotics when an alternative is not feasible, age >65, highly variable INRs, history of gastrointestinal bleeding, hypertension, cerebrovascular disease, serious heart disease, anemia, malignancy, trauma, or renal insufficiency) [7].

Prescribers should avoid use of medications known to alter INR in patients on warfarin whenever possible. Obtain INR levels in patients on warfarin therapy with suspected bleeding, especially if there has been recent addition or subtraction of a medication or herbal supplement [50].

Medications with narrow therapeutic index

Pitfall | **Failure to consider medications as a cause of vague nonspecific symptoms**

Many commonly used medications can be the cause of non-specific symptoms for which patients will seek care (see Table 13.3). A careful review of medications should be performed whenever insidious complaints do not have an obvious etiology. The following lists a sample of common medications and their adverse effects once they reach toxic levels. These medications all have a narrow therapeutic index (ratio of amount of agent that causes therapeutic effect to amount that causes toxicity) [57–60].

When toxicity is suspected, patients on these medications should have their levels checked or should be transferred to a facility with access to toxicology expertise to identify and mitigate toxicity. It is important to realize that for many of these agents, serum levels may not correlate with toxicity in cases of chronic overdose. Poison control centers can offer expertise and guidance. The national Poison Help hotline is available 24 hours every day and can be reached at 1-800-222-1222.

Herbal medicines

Pitfall | **Failure to consider the adverse effects of herbal and homeopathic preparations**

Approximately one in five adults in the United States use herbal preparations to treat illness or improve health. Herbs and their extracts contain complicated combinations of organic chemicals. It is often unknown which components of

Table 13.3 Drugs with narrow therapeutic index

Medication	
Toxic symptoms	Factors contributing to toxicity
Digoxin	
Nausea/vomiting	Renal impairment
Confusion	Advanced age
Lethargy	Hypoxia
Depression	Myocardial ischemia
Fatigue	Hypothyroidism
Headache	Hypokalemia
Paresthesias	Hypomagnesemia
Weakness	Hypercalcemia
Scotomata	
Palpitations (dysrhythmias)	
Phenytoin	
Dizziness	Acidosis
Ataxia	Uremia
Tremors	Hepatitis
Lethargy	Hypoalbuminemia
Nausea and vomiting	Valproic acid
Slurred speech	NSAIDs
Blurred vision	Amiodarone
Diplopia	SSRIs
Confusion	Ciprofloxacin
Hallucinations	Ethanol
	Pregnancy
Lithium	
Nausea/vomiting	Renal impairment
Tremor	Dehydration
Agitation	
Muscle weakness	
Ataxia	
Confusion	
Dysarthria	
Rigidity	
Tacrolimus	
Headache	Hepatic failure
Tremor	Cyclosporine
Nausea/vomiting	Calcium channel
Diarrhea	blockers
Alopecia	Antifungal agents
	Erythromycin
	Glucocorticoids
	Grapefruit juice

Data from [57–60]

preparations are biologically active in humans. Uniformity of the components is rare as several factors in the growth, mixing, and packaging of herbs cause heterogeneity of finished product.

Though widely used, there is a paucity of good quality studies demonstrating the effectiveness of herbal preparations. Data supporting efficacy exists for only four of the top 10 most commonly used herbs in the U.S. Garlic for treatment of hypercholesterolemia, ginkgo biloba to treat dementia, saw palmetto for urine flow rates, and St. John's wort for treatment of mild to moderate depression appear to have some efficacy, though the clinical importance of these modest gains are uncertain. Little or no evidence exists to refute or support efficacy for over 20,000 other herbal products.

Herbal product and dietary supplement manufacturers are not required to submit safety data to the Food and Drug Administration (FDA). However, a recent survey found nearly 60% of Americans believed a government agency approved herbs or supplements before they could be sold [61]. Direct toxic effects, allergic reactions, contaminants, and drug–drug interactions can cause serious and lethal side effects from herbs. Garlic, ginkgo biloba, and ginseng all have been shown to increase risk of bleeding during surgery. St. John's wort decreases plasma concentrations of amitriptyline, cyclosporine, and digoxin, and decreases the INR in patients taking warfarin. It can cause symptoms of serotonin excess when taken with sertraline and paroxetine [61].

Nonmedicinal products with psychotropic effects are increasingly being abused. JWH-018 is a synthetic cannabinoid that is added to herbs and sold as an incense beginning in 2009. It is known by the name "K2" or "Spice" and is becoming popular among youths. JWH-018 contains psychoactive properties and may precipitate psychosis. Emergence of this product has prompted hundreds of calls to poison control centers, and several states have, or are introducing, legislation to ban its use [62].

Awareness of the use and side effects of herbal medicines is crucial in understanding their role in treating disease states and potentially dangerous outcomes.

> | KEY FACT | Medications have the potential
> for toxicity which must be considered when
> evaluating any patient.

Pitfalls in special populations

Drugs to avoid in the elderly

Pitfall | **Failure to assess risks and benefits of high-risk medications in the elderly**

The updated Beers criteria for potentially inappropriate medication use in the elderly were published in 2003. An expert panel concluded that 66 medications were considered to have adverse outcomes of high severity in the elderly. Forty-eight medications or medication classes were identified to avoid in older adults. Adverse reactions leading to arrhythmias, sedation, falls, and anticholinergic adverse effects were common reasons for inclusion. The full list can be accessed by going to http: // archinte.ama-assn.org/cgi/reprint/163/22/2716 [63]. Whenever possible, a medication on this list should be avoided in elderly patients. Avoidance of all these medications in elderly patients may be impractical. Assessment and discussion of the risks and benefits of use of these medications must occur whenever these medications are prescribed to elderly patients.

Drugs that are contraindicated in pregnancy

Pitfall | **Failure to consider pregnancy status when prescribing medications**

Several medications have teratogenic and/or embryocidal effects. The fetus is at greatest risk of teratogenic effects during the first trimester. Drug administration during pregnancy can potentially cause congenital anatomic malformations, and can also affect social, intellectual, and functional development. Patients' pregnancy status must be considered when prescribing medications as many patients in their first trimester are unaware they are pregnant. When using agents in pregnancy, one must weigh the therapeutic benefit with the potential risk to the developing fetus [64]. The FDA issues a risk factor for each drug. Grouping into these five categories can oversimplify a complex topic. We recommend having available a more in-depth text or reference to consult when specific questions arise. In 2008, the FDA proposed eliminating the current categories and replace these with subsections on risk summary, clinical considerations to support patient care decisions and counseling, and a detailed data section [65]. Most medications lack sufficient study to provide clear guidance. An assessment of the risks and benefits of medication use in pregnant patients must occur.

Pitfall | **Failure to use a computerized support system to assist with prescribing**

Patient safety and prevention of medication errors are a top priority for health care organizations. Prevention of errors at the prescribing stage is an essential component. Prescribing problems leading to patient harm can arise from prescribing medications with potential drug-drug interactions, inappropriate doses, contraindications, allergies, or drug duplication. Failure to warn of potential adverse drug reactions can also have negative consequences. Fortunately, pharmacists often act as a "safety net" and are able to detect problem prescriptions. However, it is unreasonable to believe pharmacists will catch all problematic prescriptions. When mistakes are caught, corrective action is often time consuming for the pharmacist and may result in a repeat visit to the urgent care center. A computerized decision support system should be employed by all prescribing practitioners to reduce prescribing errors. Benefits of computerized prescribing include speed, improved legibility, and automated record keeping [66]. Decision support with warnings of clinically significant interactions or potential dosing errors are essential for preventing prescribing errors. In 2012, this industry is relatively young but with time, will develop an electronic record that improves patient safety without compromising efficiency. If computerized prescribing is not available, an electronic support instrument should be used to check for dosing, contraindications, drug interactions, need for monitoring, and anticipatory guidance for adverse effects.

> KEY FACT | **Efforts should be made to incorporate a computerized decision support system in patient care workflow to avoid the numerous and complex potential drug interactions and side effects.**

Pearls for improving patient outcomes

• The higher the generation of cephalosporin the lower the likelihood of penicillin cross-reactivity.

• Always counsel patients on potential adverse drug events.

• Avoid prescribing NSAIDs to patients at high risk for renal failure or gastrointestinal bleeding.

• Remember to calculate total acetaminophen doses in patients taking combination products.

• When administering local anesthetics, be aware of the maximum safe dose to prevent toxicity and ameliorate injection pain by using buffered warmed solution, and injecting slowly.

• Beware of drugs that could cause ventricular arrhythmia is patients with a prolonged QTc interval.

• Treat medication-induced akathisia with diphen-hydramine.

• Antibiotic restraint will prevent the risk of dangerous adverse effects.

• Avoid medications that increase fall risk in the elderly.

• Recognize that some rashes may be caused by mediations.

• Carefully select medications when prescribing to a patient taking warfarin and monitor INR closely to prevent bleeding complications.

• Recognize that medications with a narrow therapeutic index can be a cause of non-specific symptoms once a toxic level is reached.

• Beware of adverse effects of common herbal supplements.

• Know which medications are contraindicated in pregnancy.

• Use a computerized aid to assist with prescribing.

References

1 AERS Patient Outcomes By Year [Internet] 2010 Mar 31 [updated 2010 May 21; cited 2011 Apr 19]. Available from: http://www.fda.gov/Drugs/GuidanceCompliance RegulatoryInformation/Surveillance/AdvAdverse DrAdvers/ucm070461.htm

2 Xu J, Kochanek K, Murphy S, Tejada-Vera B. Deaths: Final data for 2007. *National Vital Statistics Report* [Internet]. 2010 May 20 [cited 2011 Apr 19]; **58**(19): 1–135. Available from: http://www.cdc.gov/nchs/data/nvsr/nvsr58/nvsr58_19.pdf

3 Zed PJ, Abu-Laban RB, Balen RM, *et al.* Incidence, severity and preventability of medication-related visits to the emergency department: a prospective study. *CMAJ* 2008 Jun 3; **178**(12): 1563–1569.

4 Lowell MJ. Esophagus, stomach, and duodenum. In: Marx JA (ed.), *Rosen's Emergency Medicine* (7th edn.). Philadelphia: Elsevier; 2010.

5 Innes GD, Zed PJ. Basic pharmacology and advances in emergency medicine. *Emerg Med Clin North Am* 2005 May; **23**(2): 433–465, ix–x.

6 Lanza FL. A guideline for the treatment of prevention of NSAID-induced ulcers. *Am J Gastroenterol* 1998 Nov; **93**(11): 2037–2046.

7 *Micromedex® Healthcare Series* [intranet database]. Version 1.0. Greenwood Village, Colo: Thompson Healthcare.

8 Brent J, Palmer R. Acetaminophen. In: Wolfson A (ed.), *Harwood-Nuss' Clinical Practice of Emergency Medicine* (4th edn.). Philadelphia: Lippincott Williams and Wilkens; 2005.

9 Motov SM, Khan AN. Problems and barriers of pain management in the emergency department: Are we ever going to get better? *J Pain Res* 2008 Dec 9; **2**: 5–11.

10 Todd KH, Ducharme J, Choiniere M, *et al.* Pain in the emergency department: results of the pain and emergency medicine initiative (PEMI) multicenter study. *J Pain* 2007 Jun; **8**(6): 460–466.

11 Mills AM, Shofer FS, Boulis AK, *et al.* Racial disparity in analgesic treatment for ED patients with abdominal or back pain. *Am J Emerg Med* 2010 Apr 30. [Epub ahead of print]

12 Chen EH, Shofer FS, Dean AJ, *et al.* Gender disparity in analgesic treatment of emergency department patients with acute abdominal pain. *Acad Emerg Med* 2008 May; **15**(5): 414–418.

13 Walwyn WM, Miotto KA, Evans CJ. Opioid pharmaceuticals and addiction: the issues, and research directions seeking solutions. *Drug Alcohol Depend* 2010 May 1; **108**(3): 156–165.

14 Chou R, Fanciullo GJ, Fine PG, *et al.* Opioids for chronic noncancer pain: prediction and identification of aberrant drug-related behaviors: a review of the evidence for an American Pain Society and American Academy of Pain Medicine clinical practice guideline. *J Pain* 2009 Feb; **10**(2): 131–146.

15 Sinatra R. Causes and consequences of inadequate management of acute pain. *Pain Med* 2010 Dec; **11**(12): 1859–1871.

16 Tietze KJ. Pain control in the critically ill adult patient. In: Basow D (ed.), *UpToDate*. Waltham, MA. UpToDate; 2011.

17 Groban L. Central nervous system and cardiac effects from long-acting amide local anesthetic toxicity in the intact animal model. *Reg Anesth Pain Med* 2003 Jan–Feb; **28**(1): 3–11.

18 Mulroy MF, Hejtmanek MR. Prevention of local anesthetic systemic toxicity. *Reg Anesth Pain Med* 2010 Mar–Apr; **35**(2): 177–180.

19 Catterall WA, Mackie K. Chapter 20. Local Anesthetics (Chapter). Brunton LL, Chabner BA, Knollmann BC: *Goodman & Gilman's The Pharmacological Basis of Therapeutics*, 12e: http: //www.accessmedicine.com/content. aspx?aID=16665256.

20 Hollander J, Singer A. Wound management. In: Wolfson A (ed.), *Harwood–Nuss' Clinical Practice of Emergency Medicine* (4th edn.). Philadelphia: Lippincott Williams and Wilkens; 2005.

21 McGee DL. Local and topical anesthesia. In: Roberts JR, Hedges JR (eds.), *Clinical Procedures in Emergency Medicine* (5th edn.). Philadelphia: Elsevier; 2009.

22 Christoph RA, Buchanan L, Begalla K, Schwartz S. Pain reduction in local anesthetic administration through pH buffering. *Ann Emerg Med* 1988 Feb; **17**(2): 117–120.

23 Colaric KB, Overton DT, Moore K. Pain reduction in lidocaine administration through buffering and warming. *Am J Emerg Med* 1998 Jul; **16**(4): 353–356.

24 Scarfone RJ, Jasani M, Gracely EJ. Pain of local anesthetics: rate of administration and buffering. *Ann Emerg Med* 1998 Jan; **31**(1): 36–40.

25 Barnes BJ, Hollands JM. Drug-induced arrhythmias. *Crit Care Med* 2010 Jun; **38**(6 Suppl): S188–S197.

26 Sharkey KA, Wallace JL. Chapter 46. Treatment of disorders of bowel motility and water flux; anti-emetics; agents used in biliary and pancreatic disease. Brunton LL, Chabner BA, Knollmann BC: *Goodman & Gilman's The Pharmacological Basis of Therapeutics*, 12e: http://www. accessmedicine.com/content.aspx?aID=16675372.

27 Drugs to be avoided by congenital long QT patients [Internet]. 2010 Aug 9 [cited 2011 Apr 22]. Available from: http://www.azcert.org/medical-pros/drug-lists/ CLQTS.cfm#

28 Charbit B, Alvarez JC, Dasque E, *et al.* Droperidol and ondansetron-induced QT interval prolongation: a clinical drug interaction study. *Anesthesiology* 2008 Aug; **109**(2): 206–212.

29 McKechnie K, Froese A. Ventricular tachycardia after ondansetron administration in a child with undiagnosed long QT syndrome. *Can J Anaesth* 2010 May; **57**(5): 453–457.

30 Cubeddu LX. QT prolongation and fatal arrhythmias: a review of clinical implications and effects of drugs. *Am J Ther* 2003 Nov–Dec; **10**(6): 452–457.

31 Drugs with a risk of torsades de pointes [Internet]. 2008 Mar 25 [cited 2011 Apr 22]. Available from: http: //www.azcert.org/medical-pros/drug-lists/bycategory.cfm#

32 Anon. Prochlorperazine: drug information. In: Basow D (ed.), *UpToDate*. Waltham, MA. UpToDate, 2011.

33 Vinson DR. Diphenhydramine in the treatment of akathisia induced by prochlorperazine. *J Emerg Med* 2004 Apr; **26**(3): 265–270.

34 Patanwala AE, Amini R, Hays DP, Rosen P. Antiemetic therapy for nausea and vomiting in the emergency department. *J Emerg Med* 2010 Sep; **39**(3): 330–336.

35 Linder JA, Singer DE. Desire for antibiotics and antibiotic prescribing for adults with upper respiratory tract infections. *J Gen Intern Med* 2003 Oct; **18**(10): 802–807.

36 McKay B. Caution is prescribed for antibiotics. *The Wall Street Journal* [Internet]. Sep 2003 17 [cited 2011 Oct 17]. Available from: http://online.wsj.com/article /0,SB10637512708585400,00.html

37 Welschen I, Kuyvenhoven MM, Hoes AW, Verheij TJ. Effectiveness of a multiple intervention to reduce antibiotic prescribing for respiratory tract symptoms in primary care: a randomised controlled trial. *BMJ* 2004 Aug 21; **329**(7463): 431.

38 Arroll B. Antibiotics for upper respiratory tract infections: an overview of Cochrane reviews. *Respir Med.* 2005 Mar; **99**(3): 255–261.

39 Spurling GK, Del Mar CB, Dooley L, Foxlee R. Delayed antibiotics for symptoms and complications of respiratory infections. *Cochrane Database Syst Rev.* 2004 Oct **18**; 4: CD004417.

40 Bartlett JG. Narrative review: the new epidemic of Clostridium difficile-associated enteric disease. *Ann Intern Med* 2006 Nov 21; **145**(10): 758–764.

41 Frazee BW, Lynn J, Charlebois ED, *et al.* High prevalence of methicillin-resistant Staphylococcus aureus in emergency department skin and soft tissue infections. *Ann Emerg Med* 2005 Mar; **45**(3): 311–320.

42 Petri WA. Chapter 53. Penicillins, cephalosporins, and other β-lactam antibiotics. In: Brunton LL, Chabner

BA, Knollmann BC: *Goodman & Gilman's The Pharmacological Basis of Therapeutics*, 12e: http: //www.accessmedicine.com/content.aspx?aID=16677300.

43 Apter AJ, Kinman JL, Bilker WB, *et al.* Is there cross-reactivity between penicillins and cephalosporins? *Am J Med* 2006 Apr; **119**(4): 354.e11–19.

44 DePestel DD, Benninger MS, Danziger L, *et al.* Cephalosporin use in treatment of patients with penicillin allergies. *J Am Pharm Assoc* 2008 Jul–Aug; **48**(4): 530–540.

45 Robinson JL, Hameed T, Carr S. Practical aspects of choosing an antibiotic for patients with a reported allergy to an antibiotic. *Clin Infect Dis* 2002 July 1; **35**(1): 26–31.

46 Carraccio TR, Mofenson HC, McFee RB. Benzodiazepines. In: Wolfson A (ed.), *Harwood-Nuss' Clinical Practice of Emergency Medicine* (4th edn.). Philadelphia. Lippincott Williams and Wilkens; 2005.

47 Cumming RG. Epidemiology of medication-related falls and fractures in the elderly. *Drugs Aging* 1998 Jan; **12**(1): 43–53.

48 Woolcott JC, Richardson KJ, Wiens MO, *et al.* Meta-analysis of the impact of 9 medication classes on falls in elderly persons. *Arch Intern Med* 2009 Nov 23; **169**(21): 1952–1960.

49 Hazin R, Abuzetun JY, Khatri KA. Derm diagnoses you can't afford to miss. *J Family Pract* 2009 Jun; **58**(6): 298–306.

50 Weitz JI. Chapter 30. Blood coagulation and anticoagulant, fibrinolytic, and antiplatelet drugs. In: Brunton LL, Chabner BA, Knollmann BC: *Goodman & Gilman's The Pharmacological Basis of Therapeutics*, 12e: http: //www.accessmedicine.com/content.aspx?aID=16668944.

51 Wysowski DK, Nourjah P, Swartz L. Bleeding complications with warfarin use: a prevalent adverse effect resulting in regulatory action. *Arch Intern Med* 2007 Jul 9; **167**(13): 1414–1419.

52 Hooper DC. Fluoroquinolones. In: Basow D (ed.), *UpToDate*. Waltham, MA. UpToDate; 2011.

53 Carroll DN, Carroll DG. Interactions between warfarin and three commonly prescribed fluoroquinolones. *Ann Pharmacother* 2008 May; **42**(5): 680–685.

54 Lane MA, Devine ST, McDonald JR. High-risk antimicrobial prescriptions among ambulatory patients on warfarin. *J Clin Pharm Ther* 2011 Apr 24. doi: 10.1111/j.1365–2710.2011.01270.x. [Epub ahead of print]

55 Glasheen JJ, Fugit RV, Prochazka AV. The risk of overanticoagulation with antibiotic use in outpatients on stable warfarin regimens. *J Gen Intern Med* 2005 Jul; **20**(7): 653–656.

56 American Geriatrics Society Clinical Practice Committee. The use of oral anticoagulants (warfarin) in older people. American Geriatrics Society guideline. *J Am Geriatr Soc* 2002 Aug; **50**(8): 1439–1445.

57 Kashani JS, Gerkin RD. Cardiac Glycosides. In: Wolfson A (ed.), *Harwood-Nuss' Clinical Practice of Emergency Medicine* (4th edn.). Philadelphia: Lippincott Williams and Wilkins; 2005.

58 Kearney TE. Phenytoin. In: Wolfson A (ed.), *Harwood-Nuss' Clinical Practice of Emergency Medicine* (4th edn.). Philadelphia: Lippincott Williams and Wilkins; 2005.

59 Kulig KW. Lithium. In: Wolfson A (ed.), *Harwood-Nuss' Clinical Practice of Emergency Medicine* (4th edn.). Philadelphia: Lippincott Williams and Wilkins; 2005.

60 Krensky AM, Bennett WM, Vincenti F. Chapter 35. Immunosuppressants, tolerogens, and immunostimulants. In: Brunton LL, Chabner BA, Knollmann BC: *Goodman & Gilman's The Pharmacological Basis of Therapeutics*, 12e: http: //www.accessmedicine.com/content.aspx?aID=16671319.

61 Bent S, Ko R. Commonly used herbal medicines in the United States: a review. *Am J Med* 2004 Apr 1; **116**(7): 478–485.

62 Falkowski C. Trends in drug abuse among Minnesota youths. *Minn Med* 2010 Sep; **93**(9): 47–50.

63 Fick DM, Cooper JW, Wade WE, *et al.* Updating the Beers criteria for potentially inappropriate medication use in older adults: results of a US consensus panel of experts. *Arch Intern Med* 2003 Dec 8–22; **163**(22): 2716–2724.

64 Briggs GG, Freeman RK, Yaffe SJ (eds.). *Drugs in Pregnancy and Lactation*. Philadelphia: Lippincott Williams and Wilkins; 2005.

65 *Pregnancy and Lactation Labeling* [Internet] 2011 Feb 11 [cited 2011 May 1]. Available from: http://www.fda.gov/Drugs/DevelopmentApprovalProcess/DevelopmentResources/Labeling/ucm093307.htm

66 Chen YF, Neil KE, Avery AJ, *et al.* Prescribing errors and other problems reported by community pharmacists. *Ther Clin Risk Manag* 2005 Dec; **1**(4): 333–342.

CHAPTER 14

Talking the Talk: Effective Communication in Urgent Care

Stephen M. Schenkel

Department of Emergency Medicine, University of Maryland School of Medicine and Mercy Medical Center, Baltimore, MD, USA

Introduction

Urgent care takes place in settings of constant communication. As acute care providers, we take histories, answer phones, explain options, recommend decisions, and arrange for follow-up. While doing this, we are frequently interrupted, often asked for clarification, and occasionally misunderstood [1]. Interruptions provide a nice example of the toll that normal communications can take on clinical activity and the complexity of the topic. One recent study suggests that physicians in an emergency room are interrupted more than six times an hour, returning to the interrupted task only four times out of five [2]. While the urgent care setting has not specifically been studied, there is no reason to think that it differs markedly from other outpatient areas that have received attention. Sometimes an interruption may be necessary in order to assure the safety of the patient – as when a new result suggests a diagnosis more severe than initially considered; more often, an interruption may lead to distraction, disorganization, and delay [3]. The simple solution, to make a "no interruption" rule, would not provide a satisfactory result. The obvious corollary, "interrupt only when important and necessary," is typically too vague to put into effect. In clinical practice, a keen appreciation of the pitfall may be our best approach: "Pitfall – Underappreciating the cognitive danger of interruptions."

The enormity of the field of communications prevents a comprehensive review in a single chapter. Therefore, what follows here are common pitfalls and dangers that may appear any day, at any time, in urgent care. They are arranged in the order of a typical visit: introduction and history taking, evaluation, testing and results, discharge, and follow-up. Because communication is inherently social, all the pitfalls and associated suggestions must be considered within the cultural dynamic of the department. This does not mean that the specific pitfalls don't exist everywhere; most of them do. It does mean that their understanding and interpretation should be adjusted to local conditions and norms.

Pitfall | Thinking communication does not matter

If you've made it this far, it is unlikely that we need to convince you of the importance of good communication. Just in case, it's worth considering why we bother discussing communication, much less researching it [4].

From a very basic point of view, "communication failure" frequently appears in the list of what went wrong during the evaluation of a medical event gone awry. This may be on account of the density of communication in clinical practice and points out the room for improvement [5]. Training in specific communications skills has been shown to

Urgent Care Emergencies: Avoiding the Pitfalls and Improving the Outcomes, First Edition.
Edited by Deepi G. Goyal and Amal Mattu.
© 2012 John Wiley & Sons, Ltd. Published 2012 by John Wiley & Sons, Ltd.

improve the medical student's ability to organize, manage time, negotiate, and share decision making, all potentially improving patient relations and patient outcomes [6]. Our ability to communicate, and an appreciation of its subtleties, can improve relations both with patients and with staff, making for better patient outcomes and a more satisfying career [7, 8]. Effective communication may improve patient satisfaction, bolster relationships with other providers, and prevent litigation [9].

The concept that the provider speaks and the patient hears and understands is too convenient, and simply wrong. Communication demands both speaking and listening – and confirming that what has been said has also been heard. No one likes to think that the day's effort has been lost to misunderstanding, and by reducing conflict and improving relations, effective communication leads to a greater sense of accomplishment and overall job satisfaction.

> KEY FACT | **Effective communication may improve patient satisfaction, bolster relationships with other providers, and prevent litigation.**

Pitfall | **Ignoring the "little" things**

Any discussion of communication must mention Dale Carnegie, who had another way of expressing the idea of remembering the "little" things. In a chapter entitled "A Simple Way to Make a Good First Impression" he recommends that we "remember that a person's name is to that person the sweetest and most important sound in any language" [10]. The rule here holds in urgent care as in the rest of medicine. The nature of the greeting will change according to the local culture; one typically safe approach is Mr. or Ms. with the last name. A correct and respectful means of address puts the patient encounter along the right path. This is, incidentally, also a safety mechanism. A proper introduction helps to ensure that I have not walked into the wrong room or mistaken one patient for another.

What are the other "little" things that appear to make a difference? Sitting down when talking with the patient has been demonstrated to increase the perceived length of the visit [11], suggesting that the time taken to find a chair or stool is well spent. Saying hello, shaking hands, and confirming who is in the room starts the relationship on an effective trajectory, demonstrates an understanding that an urgent care visit is both a medical and a social event, provides an opportunity to make an initial assessment of the clinical situation, and helps to make sure that no one in the room will be hearing something the patient would prefer that they don't know. Apologizing up front, especially if running late or if something else has already happened to upset the patient, can prevent minutes of subsequent explanation and hours of follow-up activity. A quick apology for a "little" inconvenience may keep it from growing into a much larger headache. Remembering good manners goes a long way toward getting the little things right [11]. Good manners also help everyone remember that the patient is at the center of the urgent care visit.

> KEY FACT | **Sitting down when talking with the patient has been demonstrated to increase the perceived length of the visit.**

Pitfall | **Failing to understand why the patient has come**

For the most part, what we see in urgent care is self-limited illness. Patients don't necessarily have to come for the urgent care visit – though they may not appreciate this – and, in general, they make a choice regarding whether or not they wish to be seen. Typically, there is a compelling reason why a patient has chosen any given time to seek urgent care. And there is always a trade-off in their decision to visit. They may have to spend money to be seen; they may lose time from work; they may simply lose time from their day.

The compelling reason for the visit may not be clear, particularly if we ignore the social aspects of illness. Much of the time the reason for the visit will be medical, such as worsening pain or a cough that has lasted longer than the patient thinks it should, and much of the time the reason will be social, such as the need for a work note. They may be seeking reassurance, a specific medication, a particular approach, or satisfaction for a family member or friend who has pushed them to seek care. Underappreciating the reason for the visit is a mistake. If the underlying reason is not understood, the patient leaves unsatisfied and the care provider may be mystified. Often, patients will shroud a social reason for a visit within a medical context. If the care provider does not ask about the social context, the opportunity for real communication may be lost. For this reason, it is essential to ask about family, job, and social needs. A few questions may prove helpful:

• What made you change your plans today to come for a visit today?
• What can I do for you that would be most helpful?
• What are you hoping I can do for you today?
• Is there something different going on at home? At work?
• Is there anything else you need today?
• Is there anything more that I can do for you today?

> KEY FACT | **The secret in caring for the patient is caring about the patient.**

Frequently, patients choose when to go to an acute care provider and what provider they see. To the degree that people have a choice, an urgent care center must satisfy the patient that their need has been met. From this perspective, urgent care is fundamentally about patient satisfaction. Furthermore, evidence suggests that the happier the patient is with the treatment, the more positively they will view the treatment, and the better they will feel. Where many of the symptoms are primarily subjective, including the pain from a sprain and the inconvenience of a runny nose, essential aspects of the treatment are encouragement and explanation [12, 13]. With this in mind it's essential to understand why the patient has come. This doesn't mean that we must give them *exactly* that. It does mean that we need to recognize the desire, respond appropriately, and potentially negotiate an alternative. In the words of Francis W. Peabody, "the secret of the care of the patient is

in caring for the patient." This is as true in urgent care as it is anywhere else in the medical world.

Pitfall | **Ignoring local news and local events**

One of the defining features of urgent care is that patients decide when they wish to seek care. Their determination of their own potential illness may be strongly influenced, however, by family, friends – and by the media. Movies, television, the web, and newspaper all convey news of recent illness among celebrities, recent events, and new medical theories that can convince patients of the need for evaluation. Celebrities frequently use this to widen knowledge of a certain illness – so we are more aware of Parkinson's disease from actor Michael J. Fox and more aware of breast cancer through the efforts of former First Lady Betty Ford.

Local news and events can be equally influential. An outbreak of illness may convince people of the need to see a physician even when they are urged to stay home if the symptoms are not severe. Within the last few years, H1N1 influenza led to overwhelmed urgent care facilities around the world as patients wanted to know the cause of their viral illness and be certain that they were not going to die from what initially appeared to be a particularly virulent flu. Even the rumor of a case of meningococcal meningitis may lead to an influx of exposed individuals concerned that they need a prophylaxis. A local case of rabies is likely, for a time, to increase the number of patients with dog bites, cat bites, and rodent bites who present for acute care.

The appearance of local physicians and hospitals in the news may also influence patients' decisions to seek evaluation. If a well-known physician or hospital appears in the newspaper for anything less than excellent care, concerned patients may seek second or third opinions, having lost their trust in the person or institution from whom they would normally seek care.

Ironically, few patients will acknowledge the role of local events in guiding them to seek care. They may describe their symptoms easily, and without any indication of what made the symptoms particularly worrisome. Only with careful observation, and with an eye toward local news and events, will the astute acute care provider be able to put it all together. A few easy questions regarding local news may put the patient at ease and assure patient and provider that the symptoms haven't changed as much as their interpretation in light of recent events. The shared understanding of circumstance both makes the diagnosis and helps to communicate its significance.

Pitfall | **Pretending money is not part of the medical relationship – and not talking about it**

Part of the decision for the patient in seeking urgent care is whether the costs will be worth any benefit received. The costs take many forms including the time spent, the effort in transportation, the explanation to friends and family, and, not to be ignored, the financial charge. How costs are calculated depends on multiple factors including the patient's insurance, the nature of the medical system, and the nature of the urgent care. Some urgent carers are quite clear, posting charges on a sign at the entrance; others hide the costs, pretending they do not exist, until a bill arrives later in the mail.

No matter the arrangement, the cost of medical care is a locus for frustration and often best handled up front. (The exception here may be those systems in which the patient bears no cost and is not expected to bear any cost.) A rise in patient complaints typically occurs when patients later receive a bill in the mail, particularly if they find the charges unexpected or notably out of line with the services they feel they received. Ignoring these costs, and pretending them away during the visit, only increases the risk of complaint and dissatisfaction.

Costs of therapy may also be too easily ignored. Physical therapy may be suggested for back pain or complex drug regimens may be written for an asthmatic, but if the patient cannot afford the physical therapy or the drugs, the treatments are meaningless. With some straightforward discussion that recognizes the limitations, an alternative approach may be readily available, for example do-it-yourself exercises or less expensive pharmaceuticals.

As if this isn't enough, the economics of medical care create trade-offs and incentives that influence the care patients receive [14]. Who owns the clinic, who is paid for research, and where costs or finances are traded among treatment groups all affect choices of therapy even for relatively straightforward acute care. In settings where market incentives are used purposely to drive decision making, the patient may have no way to see behind the curtain of decision making unless invited to look.

Pitfall | **Failing to explain to the patient what you are not doing – and why you are not doing it**

Urgent care could easily be defined as the evaluation of common problems. This brings with it a specific challenge – many patients have experienced the same problem before, or they have friends or family members who have. If not, then they may have read about the problem and potential solutions in the newspaper or on the web. For all these reasons, they come to the urgent care with preformed expectations for the evaluation and care. If these expectations match the plans for the moment, then the patient is likely to be satisfied; if not, it's a short path to a dissatisfied patient who is all too willing to place the wisdom of friends, neighbors, and family above that of the acute care provider.

If the patient actually asks a question or tells the provider what is expected, this becomes much less of a problem. But most patients won't tell. They will simply leave dissatisfied. It is our job, then, to predict what patients may want and either do it, offer it, or explain why we are not doing it. The decision of which of the three approaches to take depends on the patient, location, and practice style. For example, the middle-aged patient with one week of low back pain after exercising for the first time in a year may anticipate or even demand an MRI of the spine. Some acute care practitioners may acquiesce to such demands, regardless of the associated costs, potential for a false positive result, and guidelines advising against such practice. Others may explain to the patient why this is not necessary – then offer the study anyway. Still others may simply refuse, and explain why.

Table 14.1 Clinical conditions and unnecessary studies that patients may want or expect

Chief complaint	Studies or treatments that may require explanation	Discussion points
Headache	CT of the brain	Cost, radiation exposure, low yield
	MRI of the brain	Cost, false positive potential, availability
Back pain	Lumbar spine x-rays	Time, radiation exposure, low yield
	MRI of the spin	Cost, false positive potential, availability, low yield
Sore throat	Antibiotics	Side effects, lack of benefit, cost
Otitis media	Antibiotics	Side effects, lack of benefit, cost
Abdominal pain	CT of the abdomen	Cost, lack of specific diagnosis, time, radiation exposure, contrast reactions and nephrotoxicity
Cold / upper respiratory infection	Antibiotics	Side effects, lack of benefit, cost

Regardless of the approach, many of these sorts of expectations are highly predictable. By way of illustration, Table 14.1 lays out some of the more common clinical conditions, associated studies requested, and discussion points that help to explain why the studies may not be necessary. This discussion should not imply that these example studies or interventions are useless and should always be avoided; rather, these can be avoided much of the time and, when they are avoided, good communication includes explaining to the patient why the study or intervention is not necessary.

> KEY FACT | **Patients come to the urgent care with preformed expectations for the evaluation and care.**

How does this actually play out in clinical practice? Consider the case started above – the 40-year old male who has low back pain of one week's duration, worse with movement, better with rest, and without any neurologic signs. Before the patient has the opportunity to ask, the acute care provider can explain, "Our goal in this case is to make you feel better. Many people wonder about x-rays after a week of low back pain. While we *could* get them if you truly want, in your case I'm happy to say that they are not necessary. In general, for pain like yours, they take time, waste money, and expose you to radiation that you don't need. They would show us broken bones, but we already know you don't have any broken bones.

I recommend against them. Most of the time, back pain gets better on its own, and we'll give yours the benefit of time. While it's going about getting better, we'll work on some things to make you feel better. If the pain persists for more than a month, then we can reconsider the x-rays."

There are a few additional points worth making about this conversation. The acute care provider has removed the element of being a gatekeeper from the conversation by offering the test, then explaining why it is unnecessary. This removes from the patient's mind the idea that the provider is simply refusing. In addition, the acute care provider has offered an explanation of when the study might be necessary – after more time has passed – if the pain persists. The provider has promised to treat the symptoms which are the reason for the visit. Finally, the provider has externalized the medical thought process, freeing the patient from having to guess just what the provider might be thinking.

Even the basic language of diagnosis may change the patient's perception of necessary testing. A diagnosis of "low back pain with associated nerve pain" may not inspire a desire for radiography while a diagnosis of "sciatica" may. In a family practice, patients were more satisfied with care that omitted antibiotic therapy when the diagnosis was "chest cold" rather than "bronchitis" [15]. The term "bronchitis" seemed to imply that antibiotics were necessary. We may benefit by testing the name of the diagnosis against the planned course of therapy – and reconsidering our terms if the name implies the need for unnecessary further testing or therapy.

Pitfall | **Keeping secret when something goes awry**

In urgent care practice, significant errors are likely to be relatively rare in that most situations are simple and most patients require little testing. Despite this, there are mistakes – diagnoses are incorrect, tests are sent on the wrong patient, an x-ray finding is missed, follow-up is misplaced. In these cases, the correct approach is to let the patient know what went wrong. It can be challenging to discuss with a patient that there has been an error in care [16]. Research suggests, however, that honesty about errors is what patients want, it improves relationships, and it reduces legal costs [17]. It also forces providers to engage in self-reflection and self-improvement, resulting in improvements in future patient care and more confident practice [18]. In addition, medical ethics demands this type of honesty with the patient.

> KEY FACT | **Honesty about errors improves relationships, and reduces legal costs.**

Pitfall | **Thoughtlessly criticizing prior care**

We are our own worst enemies. In thoughtlessly criticizing another provider, we open ourselves to equivalent criticism. Effectively, we tell the patient that we do not trust each other, so why should the patient trust us. We also create an environment in which we all are open to senseless criticism, and radically increase the potential for a lawsuit.

Ironically, we are often most critical without even realizing it. We tend to forget that the provider before us saw the patient at a different stage of illness, probably before the symptoms were evident and potentially before the patient was ready to reveal the nature or degree of the symptoms. The diagnosis is always easiest after it is made; it is rarely so straightforward beforehand.

It is certainly permissible to doubt what took place before and to question the prior diagnosis. It is also reasonable to bring the patient in on these thoughts – typically with an expression of understanding that the picture of illness may have evolved since the last evaluation. Words such as "I understand why they thought this before…" or "I can see how it looked different last time around" can go a long way toward expanding trust and reinforcing a strong patient–provider relationship. The goal is always the same, to take the best possible care of the patient through all stages of the illness. Understanding that the course of illness may have changed since the last evaluation also reminds us that it may change yet again. Avoiding thoughtless criticism inspires a humble attitude that communicates to the patient the notion that the symptoms and diagnosis may change, and that the provider has the capacity to review prior decisions and recast opinions and recommendations as appropriate in new circumstances.

There is a typically obvious approach when wondering just what has happened previously – contact the prior provider, particularly if that person is a regular caregiver for the patient. Our role in urgent care is, by definition, a temporary one. If there are providers who are regularly involved, continuing care of the patient and professional relations both dictate contacting the other provider where appropriate [19]. There are often good reasons for what has come before, and the patient is best supported when these reasons are available to all providers and considered in future, and particularly urgent, care.

Pitfall | **Underappreciating the benefits and challenges of humor**

Humor in the setting of a clinical evaluation can provide instant rapport, confirming a human link between patient and provider, taking a stressful situation where anxiety limits communication to a more relaxed setting where patient and provider can speak more comfortably. It can also misfire, such as when a quick comment is interpreted as an insult or a laugh as a sign of not caring. Culture, language, and personal experience all play a role in determining whether humor can be part of a patient relationship. Omitting humor completely from the clinical environment seems soulless; including it inappropriately may be worse.

Where does this leave the individual acute care provider with regards to humor? For those who are convinced they are not funny, perhaps the approach is to omit any purposeful attempt to be funny or make patients laugh. Occasions will arise, nonetheless, where a comment leads to a laugh and a better interaction – take note of these moments and consider whether they may be generalized. For those convinced that they are funny, even comedians, pause to consider the effects of patient interactions and whether the humor has gone awry, necessitating more explanation and greater care to dig out from underneath a joke gone bad. Humor that aids the patient in understanding and coping with the acute event is to be encouraged; humor that intrudes is best avoided.

Pitfall | **Assuming that the patient understood what was said**

We often speak with the assumption that we are being heard [20]. This is true in all aspects of life, and it is particularly ironic in an acute care medical setting where pain and anxiety make it far less likely that we will be understood. The details of prescriptions and discharge instructions can all be lost in the confusion of a discharge process. Different languages, different accents, lack of education regarding anatomy and physiology, and illiteracy all work together to exacerbate the problem [21].

The first step in avoiding this pitfall is recognizing the potential for misunderstanding. Truly essential elements of care should be both spoken and written. Understanding can be best confirmed by asking the patient to repeat back, in his or her own words, what was said. A question may also lead to confirmation of understanding, for example, "So, how are you going to take this medicine?" In general, spoken or written jargon should be kept to a minimum. Patients and providers alike may prefer medical words for the idea of knowledge that they provide; patients, however, may not understand them. It is the provider's duty to translate the medical language into lay terms for the benefit of the patient, and without having been asked to do so.

Pitfall | **Failing to provide anticipatory guidance**

Pediatricians are great at anticipatory guidance; they spend years learning to predict children's futures and letting parents know what will happen, and when. The rest of us can learn from them. In adult and acute care, we also tend to know what will happen in the future, but were not as good about explaining the probable course of events to patients. For example, we know that a viral syndrome, particularly a typical viral upper respiratory infection, lasts for 2 to 3 weeks. Yet, we often give patients the impression that their illness will be better in just a few days, even asking them to return if it lasts longer, perhaps even giving antibiotics if they continue to cough. The reality is that it probably won't improve over a few days. In suggesting otherwise, we undermine our own care. If the patient believes that the cold will resolve in a few days and finds, instead, that the cough has persisted for 2 weeks, he is likely to be dissatisfied with the original care and question the skill of the clinician. More importantly, the patient may wonder about the degree to which his illness has diverged from its expected course and become concerned that something more serious is emerging – that perhaps the cough signifies pneumonia or cancer. This time the patient may demand a still unnecessary x-ray.

Patients who have experienced a minor motor vehicle collision or other minor musculoskeletal injury are in a similar position. If they come in on Day 1, we can tell them with confidence that they will be more sore on Day 2 and probably on Day 3; only after the first few days have passed will they begin to feel more comfortable. Providing them with information on the expected future course of care will let them face their soreness with confidence, potentially prevent a future visit, and burnish your own reputation for brilliance.

Pitfall | **Failing to let people know that things could get worse – and when they should come back**

The trickiest challenge in the provision of urgent care may be discovering the small number of patients among the many presenting who have a serious illness presenting subtly. While perhaps unlikely, the backache might be cancer, the headache a hemorrhage, and the dizziness a heart attack. Most patients seen in an urgent care will get well because that is the natural course of minor illness.

The greatest ally in determining whom the sicker patients might be is time. It is essential that we let patients know this, then invite them to take a part in the continuing evaluation of their illness by letting them know what to look for. If they have a cellulitis ("skin infection" would be the word to use with the patient), they should know to look for improvement in 24 hours, and to come back if it is worse after 48 hours, or if they develop a fever. Another technique is to draw a black line around the erythematous area and invite them to come back if the redness extends beyond it.

At the time of discharge, every patient should receive a set of warning signs suggesting when it is time to return "right away" [22]. This is the corollary to providing anticipatory guidance – we want to let patients know what is to be expected, and what is not. These "times to worry" should be featured prominently in discharge instructions, which ideally should be written in simple language, include the potential diagnoses, and plans for follow-up.

> KEY FACT | **At discharge every patient should receive warning signs of when to return "right away."**

Pitfall | **Forgetting to let people know if you are going the extra mile**

Most people visiting urgent care don't know what the normal course of evaluation. The only way they know they have received exceptional care is if we tell them. We should let them know what we have done on their behalf. If their regular doctor has been called, let them know. If an unusual study has been obtained – say, a necessary MRI – let them know that this is typically a hard test to get on a standard afternoon, and it was important enough that they received the extra effort necessary to put it together. For the most part, if we have not told

them that we have gone the extra mile, they have no way of knowing.

Pitfall | **Imagining the visit ends when the patient leaves**

The patient's illness does not end at the time of discharge; neither does our responsibility. The patient knows this, too. Follow-up is essential, particularly for new results or findings, such as may happen for radiologic testing, particularly if a radiologist will later read the study, or for a laboratory test that takes more time than the visit. The patient should be warned that future results may come to light and should know how those results will be communicated. Getting a phone number, e-mail address, or street address is an essential part of any visit; it allows for appropriate communication of new results.

For the acute care provider, it is equally important to be able to reconnect with the patient if something led to further thoughts later in the evening, or perhaps even led to worriedly staying awake later at night. For the benefit of one's own education and one's career satisfaction, it is essential to be able to follow-up with that patient by phone or e-mail. Call to find out what happened. There is little as satisfying in clinical medicine as finding out more of the story. In urgent care, episodic views of illness are the rule; only by following up can we obtain a longer and broader view.

We have several methods readily available to us to continue care and communication after the time of discharge. The most basic of these are discharge instructions that provide both education and guidance as well as plans for follow-up care [23]. A business card handed to the patient at the end of the encounter indicates that the provider does not view the responsibility as over; rather it is an invitation to call or follow-up. A handwritten note on the back provides an additional touch that illustrates the importance of this communication. A follow-up phone call or visit is the most labor-intensive and also the most careful of follow-up plans. Letting the patient know that he or she may receive a follow-up call or letter is an additional touch that demonstrates, at the time of care, that the relationship continues.

Pearls for improving patient outcomes

• Pay attention to the simple things – say hello, introduce yourself, sit down, and listen.

• Clarify and respond to the patient's chief complaint.

• Read and listen to local news to learn what your patients know and may worry about.

• Explain to the patient the tests and treatments you are not recommending.

• Confirm that the patient understood what was said.

• Provide anticipatory guidance and let the patient know what indicates that the illness is more severe than originally determined.

• Let the patient and family know when you have gone the extra mile.

• Provide discharge information that includes potential diagnoses, detailed treatment plans, instructions for follow-up, and information on when to return if anything changes.

References

1 Eisenberg EM, Murphy AG, Sutcliffe K, *et al.* Communication in emergency medicine: Implications for patient safety. *Communication Monographs* 2005; **72**: 390–413.

2 Westbrook J, Coiera E, Dunsmuir TM, *et al.* The impact of interruptions on clinical task completion. *Qual Saf Health Care* 2010; **19**: 284–289.

3 Rivera-Rodriguez AJ, Karsh BT. Interruptions and distractions in healthcare: review and reappraisal. *Qual Saf Health Care* 2010 **19**: 304–312.

4 Chassin MR, Becher EC. The wrong patient. *Ann Intern Med* 2002; **36**: 826–33.

5 Patterson ES, Wears RL. Beyond "communication failure." *Ann Emerg Med.* 2009; **53**: 711–712.

6 Ydedidia MJ, Gillespie CC, Kachur E. Effect of communication training on medical student performance. *JAMA* 2003; **290**: 1157–1165.

7 Murphy AG, Eisenberg EM, Sutcliffe KM, Schenkel S. The patient in 4: Framing and sense-making in Emergency Medicine. *Emergency Medicine News*; **25**: 50–53, 55. Available on-line at http: //journals.lww.com/em-news/Fulltext/2003/10000/The_Patient_in_4__Framing_and_Sense_making_in. 37. aspx. Accessed 1–07–11.

8 Cameron KA, Engel KG, *et al.* Examining emergency department communication through a staff-based participatory research method: Identifying barriers and solutions to meaningful change. *Ann Emerg Med* 2010; **56**: 614–622.

9 Stelfox HT, Gandhi TK, *et al.* The relation of patient satisfaction with complaints against physicians and malpractice lawsuits. *Am J Med* 2005; **118**: 1126–1133.

10 Carnegie D. *How to Win Friends & Influence People.* Pocket Books: New York, 1936.

11 Berwick DM. What 'patient-centered' should mean: Confessions of an extremist. *Health Affairs* 2009; **28**: w555–w565.

12 Turner JA, Deyo RA, Loeser JD, Korff MC, Fordyce WE. The importance of placebo effects in pain treatment and research. *JAMA* 1994; **271**: 1609–1614.

13 Hadler NM. The quest for a better way; or, my name is Nortin and I'm a placebo. In: Hadler NM: *Stabbed in the Back: Confronting Back Pain in an Overtreated Society.* The University of North Carolina Press: Chapel Hill, 2009.

14 Hartzband P, Groopman J. Money and the changing culture of medicine. *New Engl Med J* 2009; **360**: 101–103.

15 Phillips TG, Hickner J. Calling acute bronchitis a chest cold may improve patient satisfaction with appropriate antibiotic use. *J Am Board Fam Pract* 2005; **18**(6): 459–463.

16 Gallagher TH, Garbutt JM, *et al.* Choosing your words carefully: How physicians would disclose harmful medical errors to patients. *Arch Intern Med* 2006; **166**: 1585–1593.

17 Witman A, Park D, Hardin S. How do patients want physicians to handle mistakes? A survey of internal medicine patients in an academic setting. *Arch Intern Med* 1996; **156**: 2565–2569.

18 Wears RL, Wu AW. Dealing with failure: the aftermath of errors and adverse events. *Ann Emerg Med* 2002; **39**: 344–346.

19 Stillman MD. Physicians behaving badly. *JAMA* 2008; **300**: 21–22.

20 Makaryus AN, Friedman EA. Patients' understanding of their treatment plans and diagnosis at discharge. *Mayo Clin Proc* 2005; **80**: 991–994.

21 Clarke C, Friedman SM, *et al.* Emergency department discharge instructions comprehension and compliance study. *Can J Emerg Med* 2005; **7**: 5–11.

22 Yu KT, Green RA. Critical aspects of emergency department documentation and communication. *Emerg Med Clin North Am* 2009; **27**: 641–654.

23 Taylor DM, Cameron PA. Discharge instructions for emergency department patients: what should we provide? *J Accid Emerg Med* 2000; **17**: 86–90.

Index

Urgent Care Emergencies: Avoiding the Pitfalls and Improving the Outcomes, First Edition.
Edited by Deepi G. Goyal and Amal Mattu.
© 2012 John Wiley & Sons, Ltd. Published 2012 by John Wiley & Sons, Ltd.

LIBRARY POOLE HOSPITAL